Further praise for *Fragmented*

"*Fragmented* is a riveting, impassioned narrative that details the Kafkaesque paradox of American medicine: Despite having access to more information than ever, our doctors seem to know less and less about us. What makes it so uplifting and inspiring is that Ilana Yurkiewicz, an oncologist who has witnessed this problem first-hand, is optimistic that these challenges can be overcome—and that a more compassionate, humane health care system is within reach."

—Seth Mnookin, *New York Times* best-selling author and professor of science writing at MIT

"A lucid diagnosis of the systemic problem that has resulted in our 'broken' health care system. Ilana Yurkiewicz allows readers to see through a young doctor's eyes as the reality of fragmentation dawns during intensely emotional situations, infusing compelling narratives with humor and humanity, and making sense of inscrutable health policy issues that affect us all. Somehow, amid the chaos, *Fragmented* is able to find a glimmer of hope that is desperately needed."

—James Hamblin, MD, author of *Clean*

"From the intimacy of the hospital wards and her relationships with her own patients, Ilana Yurkiewicz tells the compelling story of the razor-thin margins by which medical care is delivered successfully in the United States, and how easily people can slip through the cracks of our health system. A must-read."

—Mikkael A. Sekeres, MD, MS, author of *Drugs and the FDA* and *When Blood Breaks Down*

Fragmented

Fragmented

*A Doctor's Quest
to Piece Together
American Health Care*

Ilana
Yurkiewicz,
MD

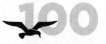

W. W. NORTON & COMPANY
Celebrating a Century of Independent Publishing

Fragmented is a work of nonfiction. The names and certain potentially identifying details of patients, family members, and health care providers have been changed.

Copyright © 2023 by Ilana Yurkiewicz

For information about permission to reproduce selections from this book, write to Permissions, W. W. Norton & Company, Inc., 500 Fifth Avenue, New York, NY 10110

For information about special discounts for bulk purchases, please contact W. W. Norton Special Sales at specialsales@wwnorton.com or 800-233-4830

Manufacturing by Lakeside Book Company
Book design by Lovedog Studio
Production manager: Julia Druskin

ISBN 978-0-393-88119-6

W. W. Norton & Company, Inc.
500 Fifth Avenue, New York, N.Y. 10110
www.wwnorton.com

W. W. Norton & Company Ltd.
15 Carlisle Street, London W1D 3BS

1 2 3 4 5 6 7 8 9 0

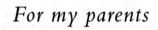

For my parents

Contents

Introduction

A FEW YEARS AGO, I WAS THE ONCOLOGY DOCTOR ON CALL when I was paged about a new patient in the intensive care unit (ICU). The patient, whom I'll call Beth Hoover, was weak—so weak that first she struggled to stand from a sitting position and later had trouble lifting a cup of tea to her lips. Next the muscles of her jaw weakened so that chewing solid foods became all but impossible. As the muscles of her eyelids became affected, she concentrated to keep them open. Finally, her diaphragm became too weak to do its job. As she gasped for air in the emergency room, her doctor had no choice. She sedated Beth, inserted a breathing tube down her throat, and connected her to a ventilator. From there Beth was wheeled on a gurney to the ICU.

I was called in because of Beth's underlying bone cancer that she had been battling for the past three years. After several kinds of chemotherapy had failed to slow its growth into Beth's lungs, her regular oncologist chose to try immunotherapy, a relatively newer class of medications that uses the body's own immune system to fight cancer. It was just two weeks after receiving her first infusion that Beth weakened to the state in which I met her: unconscious, nearly paralyzed, and wholly dependent on life support.

Could the medication have caused this? That was the question posed to me. And more important, could it be reversed? I searched the medical journals and found a handful of case reports. Paralysis like this after immunotherapy was extremely rare, it seemed, but a small number of other patients had endured something similar.

I had a few ideas for how we could treat her. We could thread a large catheter into a vein in Beth's neck and try to filter the drug out, pulling the harmful agent aside while returning the rest of her blood back to her in a closed loop. We could infuse high doses of intravenous steroids to calm her immune system, which I suspected was overreacting to the drug and counterintuitively hurting her. We could try a medication typically given to help treat other neurologic illnesses that cause weakness. Each treatment carried unique risks, with none guaranteed to work. Shortly after they called me, the ICU doctors also called the palliative care team. They wanted to prepare Beth's family for the possibility that this could be the end.

But there was one gaping hole underlying all of these possible plans: this was not the first time Beth Hoover became paralyzed after receiving immunotherapy.

The oncologist who had given Beth the medication knew paralysis was a possibility. About one year earlier, Beth received a similar drug during a clinical trial in Cleveland and became so weak she needed to be hospitalized in the ICU. But the doctor also knew that Beth had recovered completely enough for her to calmly and decisively agree to give the new medication a try.

"I promised her that if this happened again, we could treat her," the oncologist told me over the phone. "Find out *exactly* what they did in Cleveland. Then do that."

I am no stranger to working under pressure. Being a doctor requires performing effectively under the weight of extremely high stakes. I have led emergency responses to patients whose hearts have stopped pumping and have managed massive transfusions for patients bleeding out. I am accustomed to taking a deep breath, dropping everything else, and getting to work.

I confirmed with Beth's son, who was also her health care

proxy, that Beth would want to try everything possible. I told the ICU attending doctor—whose confidence that Beth could get through this flagged with each passing hour—that I needed a little more time.

The clock was ticking, only this time the situation didn't depend on how well I could do chest compressions or halt a hemorrhage. A life was just as much at stake, but it was based on a far more mundane skill—how quickly I could piece together a medical story.

THERE IS AN ASSUMPTION in an interaction between a doctor and a patient. It's so basic that it is rarely vocalized: the doctor knows the patient's story and is making decisions based on a set of information that is readily accessible. But anyone who has come into contact with the health care system intuits an understanding of medical care as fragmented, and this intuition usually manifests as a question: "Don't my doctors talk to each other?"

This is a book that will answer that question.

I am a physician at Stanford Medicine, where I practice internal medicine and oncology. From the moment I became a doctor, I prepared to face profound uncertainties because human life is uncertain. I knew that my patients' symptoms wouldn't fit textbook definitions. I knew I would puzzle over what to do about test results that landed in gray zones. I knew I'd have to synthesize high volumes of information quickly. I also knew that in the face of incomplete or discordant information, I would still have to make hard choices and act. Grappling with these gray zones was a draw for me: I was motivated to be vigilant about evidence, learn something from every patient, and develop the judgment to try to be right as often as possible.

But over my years in practice, what continues to stun me is how deeply uncertainties in medicine are compounded not only by what is unknowable but by what is simply unavailable. Medical records vanish as patients move from one hospital or doctor's office to another. Critical data get lost in a muddled electronic health file. Confusing payment practices block patients' ability to follow up with the same doctor who knows them. The result is that being a doctor means working in a constant state of being partially blindfolded, grasping at bits and pieces of a patient's narrative to try to craft a coherent whole.

I have learned to live in a different gray zone from the one I expected, applying my vigilance to patching logistical holes as often as, and sometimes more frequently than, unraveling diagnostic mysteries or communicating with compassion. I never expected it would take as much effort to find the report of a computed tomography (CT) scan as to interpret the results and decide what to do about them. I spend many off-duty hours sleuthing through disorganized patient charts. I have devised elaborate workarounds to double- and triple-check against gaps. I do these things because of a fundamental belief that the patient's story matters and that the devil of good medical care is in the details. But I also know that despite our best efforts, patients everywhere still slip through the cracks.

It has become a cliché to say that health care is broken. But the truth of this saying runs much deeper than our political and public discourse lets on. I wrote this book from my vantage point in the medical trenches, which has cemented a conviction: fragmentation—or the insertion of gaps into a patient's story, which blindfolds health care workers to the whole—is the single greatest problem underlying American health care. While tying together cause and effect is notoriously difficult in a complex field like medicine, I make the case that fragmentation's fallout is an incalculable and compounding cascade of problems throughout the entire health care system. Blood tests, scans, and even procedures are duplicated both within institutions and from one institution to the next. Vital omissions lead to missed diagnoses and suboptimal treatments.

Then there is wasted labor. In the absence of a system that reliably connects the dots, an enormous burden falls on doctors, patients, and devoted family members, all of us forced to navigate an administrative maze at the expense of focusing on sickness and healing. The data mirror my experiences: doctors spend two hours on computer tasks for every one hour facing patients. Around half of doctors report burnout, with bureaucratic demands listed as the number-one cause (this stayed true both before and during the Covid pandemic). Those saddled with the most clerical tasks are quitting, sacrificing a decade or more of expert training under the crushing weight of not being able to do their work— work with such incredibly high stakes—well. Meanwhile, patients squeeze in phone calls while tethered to intravenous (IV) poles, carry around briefcases' worth of data, and repeat their medical traumas to dozens of new faces. Those less equipped to keep their storylines straight undeniably receive worse care.

The story of how we got here is complicated. It's a story of misaligned incentives and unintended consequences. But the conclusion is not complicated: our current health care system has failed. The question now is, how do we dig ourselves out?

I CAME UP WITH A PLAN for Beth Hoover. We asked her son to sign a records release form, faxed it to Cleveland, and within the day had a stack of papers scanned into our computer system as one giant PDF. The fact that we got them so quickly was remarkable, but the hurdles of fragmentation were not yet cleared. Now was the time to dig. The records from just one hospitalization numbered about a hundred pages. Some were handwritten and hard to make out. Some were literally upside down. There were many unhelpful comments ("patient resting comfortably"), hundreds of vital signs, redundant medication lists, and somewhere, buried within, the specifics of a treatment plan that worked.

As the doctors in Ohio had done before, we set Beth up for five days of plasmapheresis—a procedure that involved removing her blood, filtering out the drug, and returning her blood back to her body. It was not easy. Beth's blood pressure kept dipping dangerously low, and we had to give her extra medications whenever she was hooked up to the machine to keep her blood pressure within a normal range. On the third day, we continued to follow the script we had unearthed by adding a steroid medication through Beth's IV at the same dose that worked in Cleveland.

By the sixth day, Beth was breathing well enough on her own that we removed the ventilator. Two days later, she stood up and stretched. Her arms were strong enough to shake my hand, and as I watched her leave the ICU, I felt like I was walking on air.

Beth did well because of medical persistence and luck, but it's all too easy to imagine how it could have gone a different way. Cases like hers bring into focus how American health care fragments a patient's story by design. I believe there are three parts that converge to create fragmentation, and I divide this book accordingly. The first part centers on data. I investigate record-keeping systems and practices that cause medical records to vanish from one hospital to another, dismantle arguments that seek to keep medical stories out of the hands of the very patients they concern, and probe the ideal division of labor to maintain those stories—not only among patients, doctors, and other staff but between human and machine. The second part addresses follow-up. This part is based on a simple premise: effective medical care is rarely a one-and-done situation. Rather, it requires an ongoing relationship: a patient must be able to see the doctor, and a doctor must be able to see her patient. I inspect an insurance system that deprioritizes follow-up in favor of emergencies; examine how twenty-eight-hour shifts—a rite of passage for doctors—fracture medical professionals into a revolving cast; and cover an innovative primary care clinic that discovered how to cultivate seamless continuity. The final part focuses on culture. I explore a medical culture that promotes quick fixes over the larger narrative, report on how the specialist's lens can splinter teamwork into silos, and ask, as individuals working in a flawed system, how we can best advocate for a patient's full story. What should doctors do, and what can patients do?

I began my medical career as a resident in internal medicine, continued as a fellow in oncology and hematology, and am now an attending physician who practices at the intersection of oncology and primary care. My job has privileged me to work in a variety of private and public hospital settings: intensive care units, hospital wards, cancer clinics, free clinics, bone marrow transplant wards, and primary care practice. While the problems I describe are those that I personally experienced, there is no doubt that doctors everywhere encounter the same systemic failures. I rotated through these different slices of health care over the years to obtain professional breadth, but doing this also gave me the unexpected advantage of seeing how it all fits together—and finding ways to compensate for the times when the pieces slip apart. Along the way, I have written about what I have observed for the past decade as a medical journalist. I do my best to blend in this book an insider's account of where we stand with a reporter's curiosity about why.

At its core, this is a book about people. Even where I change people's names and personally identifying details, I do my best to tell everything else exactly as it happened, because I believe you have to see what's happening on the ground to understand health care for what it is. I didn't seek out fragmentation in medicine; it thrust itself in my way as a recurring lesson I couldn't avoid. I learned about it while hovering over fax machines, twisting my head to decipher upside-down lab values, and grappling at midnight over whether to start urgent therapies in patients whose diagnoses trailed behind. When you confront fragmentation's obstacles this closely, you wrestle with hard questions—like the limitations of individual responsibility when the system sets you up to fail and of respecting privacy while prioritizing transparency. Tackling these questions is bound to provoke disagreement. But I come with a belief that only by making the invisible visible do we have any chance of answering the questions and fixing the problems.

THE INVISIBLE COSTS of fragmentation materialize everywhere. One spring afternoon while I was working on the hospital wards, I admitted a middle-aged man with chronic kidney disease whose left calf had swelled to twice its normal size. We ordered an ultrasound of his leg, which showed a blood clot in a deep vein, and a CT scan of his chest that showed multiple clots in his lungs. We then ordered some additional tests that homed in on a diagnosis of an underlying blood-clotting disorder that required lifelong use of the blood thinner warfarin. We started the medication in the hospital and recommended he take it continuously to prevent such clotting from ever happening again.

The hard parts were done: we clinched a diagnosis of a rare disorder and came up with a treatment plan. But fragmented medical care made the next steps endlessly harder. Warfarin requires that a patient get blood work periodically to monitor the international normalized ratio (INR), a measure of how well the blood is thinned, and then to adjust the medication dose as necessary. My hospital had a pharmacist-run clinic devoted to this task, but it couldn't take patients with other complicated medical problems such as his kidney disease. Self-sticks at home were an option, but the patient still needed someone to oversee dose adjustments and prescriptions. He didn't have a primary doctor or a hematologist, and there would be an inevitable gap until he could see one. Someone needed to keep tabs on his INR until then. But who?

We cobbled together a marginally feasible plan that called for the INRs to be faxed from the lab to the doctors' workroom, where our teams rotated every month. This plan had to account for yet another common barrier of fragmentation: most doctors' schedules involve "rotating," meaning over the course of weeks we go back and forth between different settings such as the hospital and the clinic, among many other iterations. As my rotation on the ward ended, I sat with the incoming doctor and summarized my twenty or so active patients. Then I passed along this extra task, this bizarre workaround for a patient I was about to discharge. She could have easily dropped the ball. She could have said, "That's not my job."

She didn't. For the next few weeks, the INRs for that man kept coming to that fax machine while the new doctor fine-tuned warfarin doses and called the patient with instructions. A highly trained physician was functioning as a human stopgap for a broken system, preventing this man's care from falling through the cracks.

In moments when I'm feeling particularly frustrated—when I send faxes into black holes or treat a patient once with no ability to see her again—I think of those INRs. They give me the mixed emotions I write about throughout this book: I am heartened by individual acts that go above and beyond, and I'm disillusioned that it has come to this. My work as a doctor gives me more meaning and purpose than I ever could have imagined. I take the details seriously because I take my patients seriously, and I count myself lucky to work with colleagues who do the same. But celebrating this diligence shouldn't detract from the larger, truly urgent question: is there a better way?

Part 1

The Data Dig

Chapter 1

Paper Trails

O<small>N A COOL</small> A<small>PRIL DAY IN</small> 2016, M<small>ICHAEL</small> C<small>HAMPION'S</small> wife, Leah, noticed that her husband's forehead was drenched in sweat. She took his temperature and couldn't believe the number: 102.4 degrees Fahrenheit. Over the previous weekend, he had been spending more time in bed than usual, but she had hoped he would improve. When Michael became so weak he couldn't even hold up his head, she knew this couldn't wait any longer. She called an ambulance.

I was a first-year resident working at the veterans' hospital in Palo Alto, California, when I got a call to evaluate an elderly vet with a fever. Michael was not able to tell me his symptoms. From his chart, I gathered he had long-standing diabetes. He'd also suffered a stroke several years earlier that left him with a weak right side, slurred speech, and trouble swallowing. He had a permanent feeding tube and required bladder catheter insertions several times every day. Stripped of the ability to interact the way he could before his stroke, he spent most of his time in bed or in his wheelchair. Leah was his primary caregiver.

Now she sat by his bedside, coloring in the details of a medical history he was unable to voice himself. She told me how tired and disoriented he seemed. He was pale. It wasn't right.

I ordered blood and urine tests that traced his fevers to a multidrug-resistant infection in his bladder. We treated the infection with antibiotics and worked on techniques for hygienic catheterization. Because of the infection, his blood sugar was running consistently high, so we also added extra insulin to his diabetes regimen.

He was doing better within a few days, and his mental status perked up. Every morning, when I asked how he was feeling, he was able to provide one- or two-word answers. Several times he gave me a thumbs-up.

But his hospitalization had taken a toll—especially on Leah, who now realized Michael would need to regain his strength before she could again care for him at home. He was hardly able to move from his bed to a chair without two people assisting him, and even that minor activity left him drained. The case manager on our team, a licensed nursing professional who held the job of coordinating our patients' hospital discharges, identified a skilled nursing facility nearby, just south of San Francisco, with continued physical therapy and around-the-clock nursing care. I remember Leah expressing relief about the choice. She would be able to visit him every day but could still rely on a dedicated team of professionals to help him until he fully recovered.

I performed the rituals of hospital discharge that had become second nature to me as a resident. I typed out a discharge summary outlining each of his medical problems. I spelled out his antibiotics plan. I wrote his new insulin regimen—an additional injection every six hours and extra doses with his tube feeds on top of his usual morning dose. I summarized what we were thinking, what we had done, and what needed to be done next. Whenever and however possible, I had learned to bolster that sheet. I used simple and straightforward language. I used boldface type as needed. I double-checked my medication list. I knew this sheet was often the only guidance a nursing facility would receive. If I didn't write something on the summary, the knowledge very often would disappear.

But I also knew that even if I did write all the instructions down, they might not be read by the caregivers and health care professionals who would treat him next. And I knew that only fragments of *their* notes and charts were likely to get passed down the line of Michael's care, too. And that's precisely what happened. Over the next few weeks, Michael returned to my hospital more than once, in bad shape thanks to unconnected records that were not easy to transfer.

Michael isn't alone. Every year an untold number of patients undergo duplicate procedures—or fail to get them in the first place—because key pieces of their medical history go missing. Countless others suffer from medication errors. Hospitals, nursing homes, and other medical facilities use a patchwork of methods to track records, relying on proprietary technology or old-fashioned communications such as faxes and paper notes. These systems don't always sync, and the collective costs to patients, hospitals, and the economy as a whole are impossible to quantify—although some experts say consistent and cohesive health information technology could save billions of dollars. An initiative from the U.S. Department of Health and Human Services (DHHS) aims to unify these disparate systems, but we remain far from a universal electronic medical record that would solve the problem.

Meanwhile, we have stories like Michael's, which is a story about gaps. Michael slipped through these gaps. But as I filled out his record for the first time that day in 2016, neither Leah nor I knew just how short our best efforts would fall. Back at the hospital, she and I shook hands, and she thanked me for my care.

More than a year and a half later, I asked Leah how she had felt at this point. She said, "I had my concerns about him leaving the hospital." But we had faith in the system, and she was relieved her husband would be in a skilled nursing facility, receiving help for medical problems that had become too overwhelming for her to manage alone.

He would get stronger soon, she thought. Then they'd be able to go home.

THE AMERICAN HEALTH CARE SYSTEM is dynamic by design. Patients move from one hospital to another, from a hospital to a rehab facility, from the wards to the ICU, and from the hospital to a primary care setting. These transfers are inevitable as a person's health either improves or declines or if that person simply desires a second opinion. In nonemergency situations, it's somewhat of a medical free market. Patients have every right to take advantage of it. But when the patients move, their histories often lag behind.

When I meet a new patient, I have to gather scraps of these histories from various sources—electronic records, paper documentation, outside faxes, notes in wallets, family members—to piece together a meaningful narrative. Why is this person on a steroid medication, and is there a plan for tapering? Is this poor kidney function new? How had Michael's fluctuating blood sugar level been managed when he'd been sick before?

While most hospitals in the United States today use electronic health records, they remain disparate, with hundreds of different interfaces and limited data sharing from one care facility to the next. While I was Michael Champion's doctor, only 40 percent of hospitals electronically integrated data from other hospitals outside of their system, and just 30 percent of skilled nursing facilities exchanged data outside their walls, according to the Office of the National Coordinator for Health Information Technology, or ONC, a division of the Department of Health and Human Services. A brief published in 2021 stated that 55 percent of hospitals could find, send, receive, and integrate outside patient data.

Without an easy way to get a patient's full medical files, I must ask where their prior doctors were located, have the patients sign a release form, fax it to the other hospitals, and receive stacks of papers in return. Then I dig in. Unable to use "control-find" on a stack of paper, I sift through several to hundreds of pages to find the few values of importance. If I want to see images, such as magnetic resonance imaging (MRI) or CT scans, it becomes more involved: I request the images on CDs, wait for them to be mailed over, walk them to our radiology department, fill out another form, and then wait another day or so until I can see them in the computer system. The more places the patients have gone, the more there is to unravel.

When a patient with a complex medical history like Michael's arrives under my care, it's like opening a book to page 200 and being asked to write page 201. That can be challenging enough. But on top of that problem, the middle of the book may be mysteriously ripped out, pages 75 to 95 are shuffled, and several chapters don't even seem to be part of the same story.

Meanwhile, everyone is urging me to write now.

Mere days after the Champions left, the senior resident on my team asked me to evaluate a new patient. He had a history of diabetes and stroke, and he was so tired he couldn't keep his eyes open. "Admit to medicine" the note from the emergency room had read. When I pulled back the curtain, my heart sank. The patient was Michael Champion. His frail body lay still in the hospital bed, eyes closed, and he was unable to communicate. When the emergency doctor gave Michael's sternum a brisk rub, he awoke only to fall back asleep instantly.

Leah was next to him, her face contorted. She told me that things went wrong the moment they had arrived at the nursing facility. The scheduling of Michael's tube feeds was disrupted by the antibiotics regimen. The extra insulin I had written up in his chart had also been missed.

A blood test revealed one likely source of Michael's lethargy: his blood sugar was nearly four times higher than normal. A reading just slightly higher can tip a person with diabetes into a condition called hyperosmolar hyperglycemic state, with risks of extreme dehydration, electrolyte imbalances, and in the worst cases brain swelling. Though the last is rare, its mortality rate is high. I spoke to Leah at the bedside. Incredibly, she wasn't angry. She knew it was a fixable problem, and she relied on us to fix it, just as we had his infection. But she was confused. The entire time he was in the hospital, he was given extra doses of insulin every morning, afternoon, and evening. At the nursing facility, he had been given none. How could this have happened?

Leah had hit on the million-dollar question—why?

The answer lies in the tangled evolution of e-health technology. In 2004 President George W. Bush created the Office of the National Coordinator for Health Information Technology within the DHHS. In 2009 Congress then authorized and funded related legislation known as the Health Information Technology for Economic and Clinical Health Act (HITECH) to stimulate the conversion of paper medical records into electronic charts. And indeed, many hospitals and doctor's offices did this successfully, said Karen DeSalvo, the national coordinator from 2014 to 2016 (and since 2019 Google's chief health officer), by "digitizing the care experience of every American." But each electronic health vendor made proprietary systems that weren't always compatible with one another, which made it hard for records to transfer between medical facilities. Now, DeSalvo told me, "We need to get them blended."

In 2014 DeSalvo's office had about $100 million to hit this goal. But even with this level of support, "that kind of transformation is difficult," she told me. There are hundreds of different vendors using diverse technological platforms, each with a unique way of organizing patient data. Finding a universal strategy to blend the systems has been a bureaucratic and engineering nightmare. Sometimes the barriers are intentional, DeSalvo said, as vendors don't necessarily want to make it easy to share data with hospitals using competitors' systems and may charge a fee to do so. Blocking also occurs because of a mistaken belief that patient privacy rights prohibit data sharing among doctors.

The handwringing over privacy may not be necessary. According to Lucia Savage, a lawyer and the former chief privacy officer at the ONC, the same privacy rules apply no matter how patient files are shared—whether by handwritten notes, faxes, or electronic files. "Doctors, nurses, physician assistants—they have ethical rules," she said. "They're not supposed to be snooping around someone's data because he's Steve Jobs. . . . We have to assume people act professionally and ethically in this space."

For patients the trust often already exists. When anyone comes into any health care facility, we review all the records we have. Together we openly discuss and dissect deeply personal information. In fact, patients may be the biggest advocates for sharing medical information, said Mark Savage, former director of health policy at the Center for Digital Health Innovation at the University of California, San Francisco. (He's also married to Lucia Savage.) Patients tend to take it for granted that their doctors are talking to one another, he added, and "they're frustrated when information is not exchanged."

There are data backing up these ideas. A 2014 survey of more than two thousand patients done by Mark Savage, then with the National Partnership for Women and Families, and colleagues showed that 95 percent felt electronic records "were useful in assuring timely access to relevant information by all of their health care providers." And more than three-quarters said they already share information with their health care providers all or most of the time. Those who used electronic records compared to paper records reported more trust in their providers to protect privacy.

These results resonate with my experiences. I can't think of a time when a patient complained that I or any other doctor knew too much of their medical history. Yet many times I've heard frustration that we don't know enough.

This is because the hospital or clinic is a place in which we routinely ask about and look at things that would be a faux pas at best and a violation at worst in any other context. In response, my patients don't hold back. Countless times I hear, "I don't know if it matters, but . . . ," as they bring up a bleed from twenty years ago or recount an offhand comment from another doctor. They don't ask, "Is this really necessary to share?" but instead, "What else can I tell you?" There is an unspoken contract to share more because my patients understand that everything shared is to best help me help them.

It is not that patients don't care about privacy. But people share personal, sensitive information because there is something at stake that's even more valuable to them. Trust is handed to doctors like a gift, and few things degrade it so much as patients suspecting their doctors do not know a piece of their history that is crucial to making meaningful decisions about their life. Not knowing is not just careless; it's a sign of disrespect. On the contrary, doing our homework on a patient's backstory is saying, I see you and I take you seriously. That is why four of the most reassuring words I can say as a doctor are, "I read your chart."

PEOPLE TRUST THEIR DOCTORS with their health data. But does that trust extend to others? The absence of big tech companies in the medical records saga is particularly noticeable to me thanks to proximity. I live in Silicon Valley. I can bike the 6.1 miles between my clinic at Stanford Medicine and the Google headquarters in 30 minutes. I attend conferences each year about the intersection of medicine and technology, where I am dazzled by progress in artificial intelligence that may help physicians to diagnose and treat patients better. Then I can't pull up test results from a hospital a few blocks away.

To connect large amounts of electronic health data, wouldn't it make sense to involve the industry whose job it is to connect large amounts of electronic data? The apparent absenteeism of big tech wasn't for lack of trying. In 2008, just as paper charts were going digital, Google sought to get involved through the launch of Google Health. Its goal was to create a unified health record that allowed people to store their medical data in one place. But just four years later, it shut down. According to Google, there was a lack of widespread interest among patients in the product. Privacy concerns had little to do with it. In an article covering Google Health's launch, the *New York Times* reported that "patients apparently did not shun the Google health records because of qualms that their personal health information might not be secure if held by a large technology company."

In 2018, as the scope of the problem became clear, six big tech companies—Google, Microsoft, Amazon, IBM, Oracle, and Salesforce—convened and pledged to offer technical guidance to help health care systems communicate better with one another. That year Google tried again. The new Google Health has a broader goal: to improve how health data are organized. One venture, called Project Nightingale, involved a partnership between Google and Ascension, the second largest health care company in the United States. Google wanted to build a search engine for electronic medical charts that would allow doctors to more easily wade through patient records. To give Google what it needed to create such a tool, Ascension moved its electronic health record to the Google Cloud.

Suddenly, the question of privacy was front and center. In November 2019, the *Wall Street Journal* reported that patients had not been notified. A few days later, an anonymous whistleblower wrote in the *Guardian* that because patients could not opt in, the endeavor might not be compliant with the Health Insurance Portability and Accountability Act, or HIPAA, privacy regulations. The press only got worse. The headline from *Wired* read, "Google Is Slurping Up Health Data—and It Looks Totally Legal." The *Atlantic* wrote, "Google's Totally Creepy, Totally Legal Health-Data Harvesting." CBS News announced, "Google reportedly mining millions of Americans' personal health data."

Many called Google's actions "creepy," even if legal. Most questioned the company's motivations. What are they really using this data for? They questioned whether it was done in secret, without the knowledge of doctors and patients. They questioned why it wasn't an opt-in scenario.

Meanwhile, the head of Google Health, David Feinberg, maintained that Google did nothing wrong. He responded in a blog post, saying all employees with access to protected health information went through medical ethics training and were approved by Ascension. The following year, in 2020, he spoke at the StartUp Health Festival: "The work we did with Ascension—despite what they say in the newspaper—we're super proud of." He pointed out that when you enter any hospital, your data are kept private except from third parties with which the hospital contracts, such as electronic vendors, insurance companies, and billing companies. According to Feinberg, Google is simply another third party that falls into this category. He also defended the intent of the partnership. "This is not us mining somebody's records to sell ads, to do machine learning, to develop products," he said. "We hope we can demonstrate a real improvement in care, less physician burnout, and more joy to taking care of people."

A few months later, the DHHS decided to investigate. After failing to obtain satisfactory responses from Google about how and why they collected millions of Americans' health information without their consent, Senators Elizabeth Warren, Richard Blumenthal, and Bill Cassidy sent a letter to Ascension CEO Joseph

Impicciche in March 2020. They asked, among other questions, how Ascension was planning to protect sensitive health data and whether patients could opt out.

The questions asked of Google and Ascension should be investigated and taken seriously. As efforts to exchange data go public, some critics worry less about data sharing among health care workers and more about security leaks. But a subtext of this story is that health data are not our only sensitive data; there is precedent for building data-sharing systems with attention to security. I hope Google's initial missteps become a lesson in the nonnegotiable importance of obtaining patients' consent when working with sensitive health data, not a death knell to a partnership overall. There are ways to involve third parties with thoughtfulness, respect for privacy, and compliance with HIPAA regulations. Technology companies—like everyone else who works in health care—just have to follow them.

IN THE ABSENCE of a big tech solution that reliably transmits information, we get creative. When the system fails to fill in the cracks, we hope the patients can help. I ask them multiple questions: What did the doctors say? What did the testing show? Was it a loud machine where you lie flat, or did someone use a probe coated with cold gel?

When patients don't know the answers, the burden of creativity falls on motivated bystanders—sometimes other health care providers or family members—who through grit, persistence, and clever workarounds find ways to cobble information together and pass it forward.

Michael Champion was fortunate to have a living, breathing medical record in Leah. Early on when we met, I noticed how she pulled a yellow legal pad from her purse. Later I learned that the pad accompanied her wherever Michael went, and she used it to jot down the minutiae of his care. She spoke with a deep knowledge of his medical issues, and hospital staff would often ask her if she was a doctor or nurse. No, she would say. This was a role she had acquired out of necessity.

By the time we lowered Michael's blood sugar and he was ready to be discharged for the second time, I had learned my lesson. I had performed my rituals of discharge diligently. But I needed more safeguards. When in doubt, duplicate. I devised a three-part plan: first, I would print my discharge instructions as before; second, I would call the nursing facility and verbally pass off Michael's care plan; and third, I would rely on Leah. As the only source of continuity in Michael's many transitions, Leah would be the glue. If everything else fell through, she could advocate.

Many patients don't have a Leah, though I'd seen a lucky handful who had people go above and beyond to fill in the gaps. There was the oncologist who needed the biopsy results for one of her new cancer patients. The biopsies had been done long ago at another hospital, and the patient couldn't remember who had done them or what they showed. So the oncologist cold-called all the physicians in the department; when she found that none of them knew the patient, she asked for the names of all the recently retired doctors and called them, too, until she got what she needed.

I also remember an Italian man whose clever physician spared him an invasive procedure on his heart from six thousand miles away. The man came in for abdominal pain, but the monitors capturing his heart rhythm showed ST elevations—the scary sign of a serious heart attack colloquially known as the "widowmaker." The next step after such a result is typically an emergent coronary catheterization to look for and open blockages in the heart's vessels. The patient saw the concerned looks on our faces as we watched his monitor, then calmly reached into his pocket and pulled out a folded paper that had been cut to wallet size. It was an old rhythm strip dated ten years previously, and it showed the same ST eleva-tions. His primary care physician had told him to keep it on him at all times so that any new doctor would learn he had an irregular baseline rhythm and not wheel him straight to the cardiology lab whenever he walked through a hospital door.

I thought of these stories on the morning of Michael's discharge. He was headed to a different nursing facility, about ten miles south of the first one. I spoke to Leah candidly. I told her disappoint-ing truths: discharges are the most dangerous times of a hospital stay, and I had seen plans break down even at the best institutions. Because of that possibility, I made sure she understood the details of his medical care. The nursing facility should already know these things, but if something went wrong, she could fill in the gaps.

It was unfair. Beyond dealing with the emotional weight of Michael's illness, I was asking her to carry the burden of his nuanced medical care as well. I was asking her to perform the jobs that the medical system around her was supposed to do. But no one was incentivized to care as much as Leah, and she took on the challenge with enthusiasm.

We spent the next thirty minutes talking shop. She asked ques-tions. I answered them. She took notes on her yellow sheets. We brainstormed together.

"I want to empower you to advocate for him," I said.

She put down her legal pad, reached out to shake my hand, and then, reconsidering for a moment, softly wrapped her arms around me for a long hug. She was about to head into the med-ical unknown.

THE NEXT TIME I saw Leah, she sat by her husband's side as he lay in a hospital bed again. It was one week later, and we were in the ICU. She rose from her seat when she saw me. With every visit, I swore I could see new wrinkle lines in her face. It was as though she was in a time warp, aging a year through every week of her husband's medical decline.

"It was like you were prescient," I recall her saying. "I did everything you said, and it still didn't work."

This time the problem was with Michael's tube feeds. Through his feeding tube, he was meant to receive both nutritional formula and water. Water is critical to balancing electrolytes in the bloodstream; without it, the relative sodium levels in the blood can rise. The cascade of side effects increases as the sodium level does: confusion, seizures, coma, death. But the second nursing facility hadn't given Michael the right amount of water. His sodium soared, and once again he was nearly comatose.

Leah had alerted the physician at the facility. This is completely different, she pointed out. He's not speaking. According to Leah, the response was, "This is just progression of his illness. He's a sick person, you know."

But Leah was right—though she didn't know just how sick Michael was at the time. After running a few errands, she came back to the nursing facility and found Michael being loaded into an ambulance. In the emergency room, his labs showed a sodium level nearly twenty points higher than the upper limit of normal. Michael was again in the ICU, less than three weeks after he had been admitted and discharged and admitted and discharged again. It was infuriating because it was preventable.

Leah's question was potent: "How could this have happened?" At the time, I imagined many possible answers. Maybe my printed discharge summary had gotten lost. Maybe his initial nurse left it out during a verbal handoff—where the responsibility for care is transferred from one provider to another—to be forever erased from his history.

But more likely, a nurse or doctor had held a handful of pages in their left hand and a handful of pages in their right, trying to re-create a medical story from scratch. The details of Michael's sodium management got lost in the shuffle.

In 1999 the Institute of Medicine, now called the National Academy of Medicine, published one of the most famous reports in medical history. *To Err Is Human* noted that between 44,000 and 98,000 people die in hospitals each year from preventable medical errors—a figure that was later compared to the equivalent of a jumbo jet crashing every day. While experts today disagree on their precise scope, medical errors remain a highly concerning cause of death in the United States, responsible for tens of thousands of lost lives.

In the wake of Michael Champion's case, I wanted to find data on errors that occur specifically as patients move across systems. What is the cost of these transitions? I imagined both errors of commission—of repeat lab tests, scans, and even procedures—and errors of omission, such as delayed or missed diagnoses because of an incomplete medical context.

The data we do have are unsettling to read. The Joint Commission, a large accreditor of health care organizations with a focus on patient safety, studied transitions of care and concluded that they are largely ineffective, leading to adverse events, hospital readmissions, and soaring costs. Their conclusions were supported by several key studies. One reported that nearly 20 percent of patients experienced adverse events—like Michael Champion's sugar and sodium spikes—within three weeks of discharge. Almost half were deemed preventable. And when patients are admitted to hospitals, more than half have at least one discrepancy in their medications.

How much is faulty record sharing to blame? In 2018 my colleague Marta Almli, an internal medicine doctor, surveyed the resident physicians at my hospital and found widespread dissatisfaction with how we obtain medical records: among fifty-eight physicians surveyed, four in five said it was "somewhat difficult" or "extremely difficult" to get information about patients who transferred from another health care facility. Notably, this difficulty wasn't due to a lack of know-how or effort: a majority of the same physicians said they had a "good sense" of how to get transfer materials and reported that they regularly evaluate a new patient's file when that person arrives under their care.

When the system fails, leaders in medicine suggest some tricks for improvement: better documentation, better verbal handoffs, and double-checking it all. The advice usually amounts to this: when the system fails you, be more careful—that is, work harder.

And so we do. But on a large scale, it breaks down despite our hard work. We can do every one of these steps and more, but stories like Michael's will persist because humans are fallible, memories are fickle, and it's an intellectually gargantuan task to distill decades of history in a few sentences.

We can cold-call retired physicians from distant hospitals, and we can print rhythm strips to stuff in wallets. Something relevant will eventually go missing—maybe not this time and maybe not the next. But as an aggregate, these backup plans can't be counted on as a backbone system of safety. It's also a waste of resources to rewrite a new chart every time a patient enters a new building. I've seen doctors go above and beyond in every possible way, and yet I've seen how hard it is to always get it right. As engineer and quality-control pioneer W. Edwards Deming famously said, "A bad system will beat a good person every time."

When hospitals share information, care for everyone improves. Researchers at the University of Michigan found that when emergency rooms shared files, it was far less likely for patients to have repeat CT scans, ultrasounds, or chest X-rays. Another study, this one from Israel, found that sharing health data compared to looking at only internal data cut down on repeat hospital admissions.

Slowly but surely, hospitals are venturing into data sharing. For instance, the most widely used electronic health vendor, Epic, offers a "Care Everywhere" platform, which helps facilities share electronic patient records quickly and efficiently. The company then upped the ante with a "Share Everywhere" tool, giving patients control to share some of their health data with doctors anywhere in the world. My care for veterans improved when the electronic health record system VistA (Veterans Health Information Systems and Technology Architecture) added a tab for sharing data from one veterans' hospital to the next anywhere in the country.

These are powerful steps, but we have further to go. Many experts see the last frontier as a universal electronic health record accessible across all hospitals and patients. Such a health record would transcend institutional borders. It would mean no more creative workarounds, no more paper faxes, and no gaps.

MICHAEL'S MEDICAL TEAM eventually corrected his high sodium level, and after two months of rehab, Leah finally took him home—with hospice services. Generally, in order to qualify for hospice, a doctor must certify that someone has six months or less to live. But sometimes when we cut out the aggressive medical care, amazing things happen. Some people live longer.

Such was the case with Michael.

On a windy afternoon in January 2018, nearly two years after I first met the Champions, I saw them once more, this time at their home. Michael was doing well, considering what he'd been through. Leah had decided to look after Michael's insulin and water additions herself, and she also had nursing aides visit the home four days a week. In the end, she trusted herself most. She was the pillar of continuity Michael needed—one that many others do not have.

During my visit I told Leah that I never found out exactly where the breakdown in communication happened at the nursing facilities nearly two years before. I retraced their steps and paid visits to both, trying to re-create their story. Along the way, I found no electronic trail of Michael's stay. There were some records, but those for discharged patients were filed in a paper binder in a separate storage facility.

At one of the nursing facilities, I sat with the admissions coordinator as she ran me through the intake process. How they obtain records depends on where the patient is coming from, she explained. Some places send electronic forms, and some go through fax. What arrives is a standard set of papers: the physician's discharge summary and the most recent medication list. The nursing facility doesn't receive a full set of lab values—unless the physician copies them into the discharge summary—or any notes prior to the hospitalization, such as primary care records.

I wish finding the hole was simple: a broken fax machine or a paper chart that ended up on the wrong desk. But when the process is roundabout, requiring multiple steps and multiple workarounds, the breakdown points multiply. It's remarkable that things turn out well so much of the time given all the places they could go wrong.

Michael had more fortitude than almost anyone I've met. He recovered again and again—sometimes because of, and sometimes in spite of, his medical care. But six months after my visit, in July 2018, Michael died—on his own terms. He'd had pneumonia, and it was showing signs of coming back. Leah asked if he wanted to treat it or allow nature to take its course. "His gift to me was clarity," Leah told me later. "I didn't have to make the decision for him." Michael's last words to Leah had been, "Let it go." She brought in family and friends to say their goodbyes. Then they stopped his tube feeds.

Since then I've thought back to my last visit with Michael, when Leah asked if I'd like to talk to him privately. When we were alone, I asked him, "Are you happy?"

Michael looked out the window and then turned back to me.

"Yes," he nodded.

I nodded back, reflecting on what it was like to reconstruct the entire human narrative of Michael Champion from a handful of scattered, disconnected fragments. As I looked at him, I saw all my patients, and I thought of how to get them the informed medical care they so deeply deserve. I eagerly await the day when a universal electronic health record might connect the dots. But it's not yet that day, so we in the health care system must do everything in our power to deliver good care to those who trust us with it. We will continue to push papers through fax machines, to wait on hold as we cold-call those who may provide answers, and to repeat tests from scratch when we're stalled.

We know it's not a perfect system. We know there will be gaps. But what choice do we have?

Chapter 2

Who Owns the Story?

LEAH CHAMPION RELIED ON A YELLOW LEGAL PAD TO TRACK her husband's saga. For a woman I'll call Sarah Leary, a thirty-four-year-old engineer with breast cancer, it was binders. The day I met her, on a warm Tuesday afternoon in 2018 in the Stanford Medicine Cancer Center, she had four. The red one was labeled "Radiology and Pathology," the white one "Treatment," the orange one "Labs," and the blue one "Other Medical History."

Sarah kept the binders in a briefcase she lugged from doctor's appointment to doctor's appointment. "Going back to work after this?" I had asked upon seeing it. No, actually—everything in the briefcase was for me.

Sarah came prepared. So did I. Before we met, I sat at a computer in the doctors' workroom and started my note in her chart. I wrote a timeline—beginning the moment she noticed the lump in her breast while showering—and then pulled up every piece of data I had thereafter. My goal was to write a coherent, chronological medical story.

It took about half an hour. I collated information from her electronic chart, including scanned PDFs from other doctors' offices. Even after plenty of searching, there were still plenty of gaps. Whenever I came across a narrative hole I wanted to ask Sarah about, I marked my note with an asterisk.

From the chart I learned that after Sarah noticed the lump—

firm, immobile, and creeping into her armpit—she called her family doctor. The doctor ordered an ultrasound, which showed a dark lesion with irregular borders. Sarah was sent to a radiologist who numbed her with lidocaine and inserted a needle to biopsy the mass and a nearby enlarged lymph node in her armpit. Results showed invasive breast cancer.

Next came a mammogram and MRI of both breasts and a positron emission tomography (PET) scan of Sarah's whole body. Fortunately, the cancer hadn't spread beyond the nearby lymph nodes. Sarah also underwent genetic testing to see if there was a reason she developed this cancer at such a young age. She spat into a test tube, packaged the tube in a small cardboard box, and dropped the sample in a mailbox. Next she had a port surgically placed under the skin of her chest and an echocardiogram taken of her heart. A local oncologist started her on a chemotherapy regimen consisting of three drugs infused through her port every two weeks.

But the mass in her breast did not shrink as intended. It was growing.

Sarah had come to our clinic for a second opinion. When we met in the exam room, I ran through my asterisks. Before I get to the most important questions that patients ask—What are my chances of cure? What do we do now?—I must do the meticulous, unglamorous work of getting the story straight.

"I saw you had genetic testing," I said, "but I don't have a copy of the results."

She flipped through the orange binder and pulled it out. I typed the results into the computer as she waited patiently, and then I handed the papers back to her.

"I also had a question about the most recent MRI," I started. She opened the red binder and located it.

We volleyed back and forth for a bit. My questions were in the medical weeds, but Sarah was right there with me. All of my asterisks were addressed, and I felt confident that I understood her story. Now we could turn our attention to what really mattered: what should we do about this cancer?

"Thank you for being so organized," I said, finally turning away from the computer to face her.

Any discussion of a universal medical record has to go beyond data sharing among doctors. There's another person in this equation—arguably the most important one. Yet in one of the cruel ironies of our fragmented record-keeping system, even as patients are forced to bear the responsibility of maintaining continuity in their care, they are actively obstructed from doing so. To obtain the contents of those binders, I later learned, Sarah didn't just navigate red tape. She also navigated attitudes from the medical community about what patients should see, when, and how.

As patients like Sarah traverse obstacle courses to access their own medical information, progress depends as much on syncing technologies as it does on wrestling beliefs about privacy, transparency, and ownership. These attitudes are divisive. They're also evolving. And they boil down to a basic question: to whom does the medical story belong?

For Sarah, who didn't understand why I was thanking her, the answer was obvious. "It's my life on the line," she said.

IF WE WENT BACK a few decades, my interaction with Sarah Leary would never have happened. Historically, patients were not expected to play a serious part in their own medical care, much less peek at their charts. A patient's role was to ask for help and then graciously accept what was offered. That Sarah knew her own cancer to the level of detail an oncologist asked for—and that I counted on her to know this—is telling of a relatively recent shift in norms.

By the time I became a doctor, the old paradigm had fortunately evolved. I was taught to practice shared decision-making, an approach where doctors and patients work together to choose what comes next. Whenever possible, we pull up chairs and sit at eye level rather than hover over someone lying on a gurney. We learn to be sensitive to the power dynamic inherent in the interaction between a person wearing the long white coat and one wearing a gown. It's part of our job as doctors to create safety within that dynamic, proactively and deliberately.

In turn my patients research their symptoms on the internet and have ideas for what could be going on. They bring me articles. They question recommendations. Sometimes they say no. A good doctor welcomes this discussion, understanding it is about the patient, not the doctor's ego. A good doctor encourages second opinions, engages with concerns, and is transparent in answering questions, including admitting when she doesn't know.

This is all a cultural move in the right direction. But the day-to-day practice of medicine can allow even the best intentions to slip. As a senior resident, I once supervised a diligent medical intern I'll call Andy, whom I appreciated most for his attention to detail. I could sleep at night knowing orders would be in, calls followed through, and any changes in patients' status communicated with me. One of the first patients we discharged from the hospital together was a seventy-two-year-old we admitted for vague neurological symptoms that quickly evolved into concerning ones: her left pupil became dilated as one side of her face went numb. We ordered an urgent head CT scan and saw the culprit. An artery had burst, causing a hemorrhagic stroke.

Over the next few days, we stabilized her and coordinated many services she would need for recovery. As the patient's discharge neared, I appreciated the thorough hospital summary Andy wrote. It included everything that had happened and a bullet-point list of what needed to be done next. He faxed these records to the patient's primary care doctor.

There was only one thing Andy forgot to do. "I had a *stroke?*" the patient asked during my rounds the morning of her discharge. Her eyes darted around at the various members of our medical team for an explanation.

As bizarre as this sounds, Andy's lapse was not unique. It was also not done with any ill intent. In no part of Andy's calculus did he think, consciously or subconsciously, that our patient shouldn't know that a collection of blood the size of a golf ball in her brain equated to a stroke. He plumb forgot to explain it. Andy was busy. He worked hard outside the patient's door to coordinate the care she needed. But keeping a patient in the loop fell to the bottom of the to-do list if it made the list at all.

By the time I became a senior resident, I saw that forgetting to keep patients informed—when the plan changed, when a new order was placed, or even when they had a serious diagnosis—was such a common oversight that counteracting it became something I actively taught new doctors, as high on my priority list as how to treat a heart attack or evaluate critically low blood pressure. My teams got in our daily step counts as we went from hospital room to hospital room updating our patients. Before we sent anyone home, we printed out clear instructions and handed over reports of scans and lab values. We gifted our patients copies of their hospital summaries like Santa Claus. "The patient is the only guaranteed source of continuity in their own care," I would say. My goal was for our patients to have the same knowledge of their medical story that any doctor would have. Unfortunately, there would be more than forgetfulness getting in the way.

Do patients have a right to read their medical charts? Legally, the answer is easy. In twenty-one states, the law says that medical records are the property of the hospital or physician. (The other

states do not have specific laws designating medical records ownership; only New Hampshire explicitly says medical records belong
to the patient.) However, the laws nationwide are equally clear that
patients should be given access to copies in a timely manner and
at a reasonable cost. Since 1996 the HIPAA Privacy Rule has provided people with a legal, enforceable right to inspect and receive
copies of their medical records on request (with some exceptions,
such as psychotherapy notes).

How this plays out in the real world is a different story.

Carolyn Lye was a dual medical student and law student at Yale
University in 2018 when she and her mentors had an idea: she
wanted to understand what patients experience when trying to
obtain their medical records. Lye is well versed in the federal regulations that encourage patient involvement in their own care. In
fact, her inspiration to go to law school when she was already
enrolled in medical school came from a conversation with one of
the drafters of HIPAA. But the revelation that these recommendations might be failing in practice didn't come until one of her
medical school rotations, when she cared for a patient who was
hospitalized for a week and then asked for a full set of records. Lye
realized this was harder than it sounded, as there were no standard
procedures in play to make it happen. "If I were a patient, I would
want to know what happened," she told me over the phone. "It
seemed strange to me that there were so many barriers in place to
prevent patients from getting records, when it's something they
have a right to receive and could benefit from."

Take Sarah Leary. I learned that filling those binders was a process that took relentless phone calls and follow-ups. She was grappling with her mortality. She was adjusting to a new life consumed
by infusion center visits, oncology appointments, blood work, and
chemotherapy that caused hair loss, fatigue, and nausea. But she
knew that her chances of getting through this depended as much
on her doctors knowing the details of her story as on the che-

motherapy drugs running through her veins. With something as crucial as her life at stake, she would leave nothing to chance. She told me that she would call the records departments while she was hooked to an IV pole receiving chemotherapy. This was a logical place to do it, she explained: she was trapped anyway.

Lye wanted to understand if jumping through hoops like this was the norm. She took the idea to her mentors at Yale, Harlan Krumholz and Howard Forman, and together they came up with a plan to find out: Lye would pose as someone looking for her grandmother's medical records. She teamed up with an undergraduate student to call the medical records departments of eighty-three top-ranked hospitals in twenty-nine states. They asked each hospital detailed questions about how they could obtain their "grandmother's" records: What was the process? Could the records be emailed? Was it free? What was the wait time?

When they tallied the results, a dismal picture emerged: not only were there large discrepancies among institutions; there was wide noncompliance with federal standards. The records offered were piecemeal, delayed, and costly. For two hundred pages of records, for instance, Lye was quoted costs ranging from free to $541.50. The federal recommendation is a flat fee of just $6.50 for an electronic copy of a report. But 59 percent of hospitals named costs that were higher. "The prices were outrageous for some of the hospitals," Lye said.

Federal regulations also say that medical record requests must be fulfilled within thirty days of receipt (with the possibility of a single thirty-day extension) in the format requested by the patient. But the list of options Lye was offered frequently differed from what the hospitals' websites said they could do. One hospital told her that receiving older records could take up to two months—not including the extension. In a 2019 follow-up study that examined how patients receive radiology results, Lye and her coauthors found that eighty hospitals said they could provide results on CDs; however, only 8 percent of those hospitals could offer results through email, and only 4 percent offered results through an electronic patient portal. The problem is one that was quickly identified by an eighty-year-old patient of mine when I asked her to bring me a copy of her hip X-rays: "Who still uses CDs?"

I asked Lye if it was possible that the records departments misspoke and that the institutions identified as deficient in the study actually did provide the records within the legally prescribed time and for the recommended fees in practice. "I don't think there is an excuse for hospitals not to provide patients with the right information," she said plainly. Even as I asked the question, I knew her findings did mirror the real world. I wasn't surprised by them. Patients have often asked me for printouts in the middle of clinic visits to avoid dealing with the records departments after the fact. They have told me horror stories about redundant phone calls, confusing bureaucracy, and forms lost in the mail. Patients are Odysseus, traversing a sea of obstacles just to get what is rightly theirs.

Spurred by desperation and frustration, some have tried to bypass hospitals' medical records systems altogether by generating their own. I spent one Sunday evening searching for these so-called personal health records and downloading a handful of apps with the highest ratings onto my phone. One advantage of the apps was that some let me add health information not stored in a doctor's file, such as recordings of my sleep or mental health. But as I looked up and typed in the dates of my last tetanus booster and when I had my wisdom teeth extracted, I gave up. This was manual data entry. Not only was it completely separate from the medical chart my doctors had; it was also all on my word. The information I would look for as a doctor—pathology reports, scan results, lab values over time—only existed if I wrote them in from scratch. For example, knowing that you had something biopsied five years ago and it turned out to be "benign" is helpful, but even more helpful are the details. Was it a fibroadenoma? A benign phyllodes tumor? A patient often has no way of predicting which details I would find important.

The apps also felt like they catered to a very specific demographic. The person who could fill these out would be generally healthy, with only a handful of things to track. This person would also be organized and relatively high-functioning, able to navigate data entry on a phone app. Both facts point to a certain irony: the person who could fill these out the best would likely need them the least.

In an era of shared decision-making, you would think the medical community would embrace with open arms a technological upgrade to record sharing with patients. But there is a philosophical undercurrent to the question of who owns the medical story, and the waters turn murky when a real solution becomes possible. Patients have a right to see their records, sure, but can they really handle reading what doctors write about them?

One afternoon in 2015, I sat in the doctors' workroom amid a grumble of chatter about all the ways releasing our notes to patients would be disastrous. My medical center was about to launch "OpenNotes" in primary care and the cancer center—an initiative that had started five years earlier at Beth Israel Deaconess Medical Center, a teaching hospital of Harvard Medical School. Bypassing the tortuous odyssey through medical records departments weeks or months after seeing their doctor, patients would instead be able to pull up doctors' notes on their home devices immediately after we signed them into the electronic chart.

OpenNotes was built with an opt-out function, meaning doctors could choose not to share any given note with one click of a button. But the mood in the workroom was still sour. I remember one colleague complaining about patients with chronic pain she coded in her note as "psychologic" in origin. Imagine a patient reading that? Another colleague was concerned that patients would quibble over minor inaccuracies. Would he be inundated with messages correcting him, saying that actually it was four days of coughing, not three?

I admit that I joined in. I skimmed my recent notes, wincing as I imagined my patients reading some of them. One was about an elderly woman with end-stage heart failure who I had recommended see a palliative care doctor. My explanation in the note read "prognosis guarded." A second concerned a young man to whom I was prescribing PrEP, a medication that prevents contracting HIV. I had charted the reason as "high-risk sexual behavior." A third described an encounter with a middle-aged woman who had been experiencing shortness of breath with exercise ever since having part of her lung removed for a tumor nearly a decade ago. I had run a litany of additional tests that showed no other problems, so in response to her breathing complaints I had written "no further workup indicated." Even that gave me pause. Would she read that as dismissive? Would the others read theirs as judgmental?

My notes are a straightforward blueprint of my thinking and plans. I write them for an intended audience of other health care providers and my future self. My notes are not flowery. ("Aren't you a writer?" a colleague once asked me upon reading one of my terser notes. I don't think it was a compliment.) I also don't write them with reassurance in mind. In person, if I suspected a low likelihood of cancer, for instance, but couldn't yet rule it out while a biopsy was pending, I would choose my words carefully. My notes provide no such qualifications. I wondered if reading them could undermine the nuanced conversations I was so careful to have with my patients face to face.

Our objections echoed those that Tom Delbanco—a primary care physician at Beth Israel Deaconess, professor at Harvard Medical School, and cofounder of OpenNotes—heard five years earlier, he told me. When he first made his case in a journal opinion piece, one doctor wrote to the editor castigating the "young whippersnapper" who didn't understand medicine. (Delbanco was delighted to find out he was actually ten years older than the letter author.) Undeterred, Delbanco and cofounder Janice Walker, a nurse and now associate professor of medicine at Harvard and Beth Israel, proposed the idea to primary care doctors. Many refused. Sharing their notes would confuse or upset their patients, they argued. In contrast, when Delbanco and Walker asked patients if they'd be interested, nearly *all* thought it was a good idea.

Some doctors agreed to try, however, and in 2010 Delbanco and Walker launched a small pilot in three clinics, in Boston, rural Pennsylvania, and at a safety net hospital in Seattle. After one year, they handed out follow-up surveys. Almost all the doctors reported that their workloads were the same. The patients were thrilled. At the end of the pilot, 99 percent of patients wanted OpenNotes to continue, and not a single doctor chose to stop.

This sequence of events could have been instructional for me and my colleagues, but when OpenNotes came to our hospital system in 2015, we bellyached all the same. Soon the next part of the pattern repeated itself, too: I found that not only did my notes not upset my patients; sharing them helped catch meaningful errors. Shortly after we launched, a patient informed me that my note showed she had a history of rheumatoid arthritis. But she didn't: it was a family history of the illness. Other patients, I sensed, came more prepared. It reminded me of the "flipped classroom" model that some educators use, where students are expected to learn the basics on their own so that time together in the classroom can be devoted to higher-level discussion and working through misunderstandings. All the while, the deluge of fearful and nitpicking messages never came.

"We"—meaning doctors—"don't deal very well with change," Delbanco told me. "No one does, but we do it particularly badly."

In the years following Delbanco and Walker's initial experiments, the OpenNotes movement spread to other hospitals across the United States. In 2020 more than fifty million patients in the United States and Canada could read their doctors' notes. But despite this progress, it wasn't the norm. After I spoke to Delbanco, I looked at my visits to my own primary care doctor and specialists since OpenNotes had launched at my medical center. Out of eighteen appointments, only two notes were shared with me.

When the medical community stalled, the government stepped in. The 21st Century Cures Act, signed into federal law in 2016, was given to the Office of the National Coordinator for Health Information Technology to ease the regulatory burden of patients' accessing their medical charts. The ONC Final Rule, requiring that health care systems electronically release medical records to the patients they concern, was implemented in April 2021. I last spoke to Delbanco in October 2020, several months before the mandate went into effect. How would doctors react?

"There will be 'oy veys' like you've never heard in your life," he predicted. "But they'll get over it."

THE ONC FINAL RULE took the debate over patient access one step further; this didn't involve instantaneous release of only physician notes but also raw data. Once patients created an online account, they could automatically see things like blood and urine test results, written results of CT scans and MRIs, and biopsy reports. Loved ones at the bedsides of ICU patients could view the avalanche of data we typically generate when patients are critically ill; patients in the clinic could see whether the new biopsy was benign or malignant, even before their doctors; cancer patients could review CT scans that would tell them whether the chemotherapy had succeeded or failed to halt the spread of disease.

Controversy followed along predictable party lines. Many doctors publicly and privately bemoaned the anxiety that would stem from patients seeing test results they wouldn't be able to interpret. Meanwhile, many patients celebrated the release of what was rightly theirs and condemned these outdated, paternalistic attitudes.

When the Final Rule went into effect, I had used OpenNotes long enough to welcome the changes. I was optimistic about the electronic upgrade from a convoluted workflow that had me torquing my computer screen to show patients their test results. As a handful of patients began to message me about abnormal results, another unexpected benefit revealed itself. Between my practice managing about one thousand patients and a software system that buries important results, I am always swimming in patient data to review. Missing something important is one of a doctor's greatest fears. Knowing that my patients would be looking simultaneously felt like an additional check and balance: if something was seriously off, I trusted they'd ask me about it.

The timing of release posed a tougher question. Immediate release seemed to disregard the possibility that test results could be emotionally fraught and would benefit from a doctor's explaining them. Among the many cancer patients and survivors I treat, for example, the anxiety caused by getting results of CTs and MRIs is so common that many dub it "scanxiety." Doctors asked about invoking a waiting period to give the doctor and patient time to discuss results before patients could view everything on their own. Surely a short hold to allow the doctor time to review the data and counsel the patient would not be considered a type of "information blocking" the ONC Final Rule was intended to dissuade. The most extreme camp of patient advocates pushed back: people should be able to absorb news on their own terms. Getting medical information on a personal device could liberate patients from dependence on the doctor's schedule and his or her style of delivering bad news.

Ultimately, the ONC did give leeway on the exact timing of data release, and individual clinics came up with their own rules. Mine decided to implement wait times on certain results, a decision that quickly proved advantageous. One of my patients is a woman who was in remission after completing a long course of treatment for breast cancer. A CT scan in the midst of her cancer journey incidentally found two small nodules in her lungs. These are often benign but need to be monitored. I ordered another scan one year after they were discovered to make sure they appeared stable. One Thursday afternoon, she messaged me. She was home from having the scan: when could she learn the results?

The radiology report popped up in my inbox. The default release date to the patient was in two weeks, but I could choose to release it sooner. I didn't. Instead I forwarded it to my medical assistant and asked her to arrange a video appointment with my patient for the next day.

I did that because my patient's scan was puzzling. The lung nodules looked to be stable, but her spleen was mildly enlarged, as were the lymph nodes in her chest. The radiologist had commented in the report, "Could be seen in the setting of a lymphoproliferative disease, such as chronic lymphocytic leukemia." I didn't like to imagine my patient simply reading that result before having a conversation with me first.

We met on video the next day, a Friday afternoon. I asked how she felt. Not great, she admitted. For the past week, her gums had been swollen, and she was sweating at night. She blamed it on stress.

As I listened, my heart sank. I explained the scan results and said that enlarged lymph nodes could sometimes be seen while the body battles an infection, such as a virus. However, we couldn't rule out a new cancer. We needed additional tests. I placed orders for basic blood cell counts, electrolytes, and a test called flow cytometry that could help diagnose and distinguish blood cancers.

She understood. She promised to go to the lab and get her blood drawn first thing Monday morning.

When Monday morning rolled around, I muttered a few expletives as my phone buzzed with alerts. The lab informed me that her blood counts were critically low. Her electrolytes and kidney function numbers suggested tumor lysis syndrome, a condition that can occur with acute leukemias and lymphomas in which the cells break open. I knew this wasn't a viral infection. It wasn't even chronic leukemia as the radiology report suggested. This was an acute, aggressive blood cancer.

The waiting period for blood work release in my clinic was only one hour. This time, if I wanted her to hear it from me, I'd have to move fast. I made three phone calls. First, I called her. I told her I was worried this was leukemia, and she needed to go to the emergency room. Next I called the emergency room to alert them of her impending arrival. Finally, I contacted the inpatient leukemia doctor on call to give the team a heads-up about my diagnostic suspicions and prep them to admit her for the next steps of the workup.

I am grateful for the wait times that allowed this devastating turn of events to unfold as smoothly as it could have. I was not alone. Months later, with a shaved head and her second cancer in remission, my patient told me how much she appreciated those early steps: "I always feel better when there is a plan," she said. "It was like, all of a sudden I had leukemia, but I was secure because there was a clear plan." I could not have come up with that plan without keeping my patient's CT scan hidden—not for a year, not for a month, but for twenty-four hours as I worked behind the scenes.

We can and should debate the details. Should a doctor be given seven days or fourteen days to review CT scans? Are some blood test results just as fraught as radiology reports? Should there be a difference in wait times based on whether a patient is seen in the clinic or is hospitalized? As we parse the answers, I don't see implementing brief wait times as disrespecting a patient's right to receive information but rather as a way to support the counseling part of the doctor-patient relationship to work as it should.

Even as we debate these nuances, the broader lessons from OpenNotes and the Cures Act Final Rule have been clear. The cycle will no doubt continue to repeat itself, with the next reveal of patient data provoking the same outcry: patients will not understand; patients will have anxiety; patients will bombard doctors with trivial questions. When this happens, we will continue to debunk these myths. Imposing logistical hurdles that take a herculean effort to overcome amounts, in effect, to restricting information—and restricting information is never the answer.

As PATIENTS ACCESS their medical records, a final question to contend with is not one of owning but of taking ownership. Even with technological upgrades that sync records, there will always be some level of responsibility required to keep on top of an ongoing medical saga. Without clearly defined roles, this work ping-pongs between doctors and patients and, unsurprisingly, can fall apart altogether.

So whose job *should* it be? Who ought to be the keeper of the medical story?

Here's a thought experiment. Imagine you're a primary care doctor, and the next patient on your clinic schedule is a sixty-five-year-old man named Jim who splits his time between where you practice in California and where his daughter and grandchildren live in Connecticut. He recently returned from another trip, and he tells you that his time with family was sadly interrupted by time in the hospital. Jim had pneumonia, which was treated with a few days of antibiotics and luckily resolved without complications.

You click through his chart and remind yourself that about three months earlier you had treated him for pneumonia. Actually, this was his third bout of pneumonia in one year.

A red flag waves in your mind: recurrent pneumonia in the same part of the lung can signal an underlying obstruction such as a tumor. And Jim has some risk factors, including his age and a smoking history, though he assures you he hasn't touched a cigarette in years.

You ask more about this last bout. Was the pneumonia in the left lung? Even more precisely—was it in the upper or lower lobe? Jim has no idea.

What do you do? Twenty minutes have now elapsed. Your next patient is waiting in the room next door. You have three options.

1. *You can add tracking down Jim's X-rays to your to-do list: have Jim sign a form authorizing release of records, fax it to the other hospital, call over to close the loop, wait to be connected to medical records, and wait for radiology reports to be faxed to your office. This would all be done on your own time, of course; your schedule does not permit these extra steps in your back-to-back booked clinic.*

2. *You can put it on Jim. You ask him to make the calls, obtain the radiology reports, and bring them to your next visit.*

3. *You can order a CT scan to rule out a tumor anyway. You can decide you have enough information, even if it's imperfect, to make a decision. You weigh the radiation risks of a CT scan against the administrative burdens of getting the full story.*

Do you fight for every detail? Or just move on with what you have?

Doctors constantly make risk-benefit calculations. We face many high-stakes decisions throughout a workday; there are also countless other instances of smaller decisions, the weight of which may not be apparent in the moment. One of medicine's secrets is how deeply our choices are influenced by the availability of resources, timing, and ease of administration as much as medical need.

With Jim, who is based on a real patient of mine, I chose option 3. I ordered the CT, which fortunately came back clear.

I told this story to a friend, another doctor, over dinner one night. She shook her head midway through. "Would you go to your accountant without your W-2?" she pressed me. "Or see your lawyer to review a contract—but not bring the contract?" For her it's a matter of consistency: if we're all about empowering patients, we must also expect personal responsibility over maintaining the narrative. This attitude jibes with how doctors say we should treat patients—with respect, not paternalism.

I thought about this. "Some of my patients can't do it them- selves," I said. Sarah Leary represented one end of the spectrum. On the other was a patient I thought of then, a ninety-two-year- old navy veteran. He had lost his left leg to an above-the-knee amputation after a lifetime of uncontrolled diabetes had destroyed its arteries. He was legally blind in both eyes. He had mild cogni- tive impairment that caused memory problems. His medical issues were masked by a delightful personality. Every visit he would wave at me and say, "I can't see much, but I see my favorite doctor!" He lived with his twenty-five-year-old grandson, who helped with medications and appointments but who also had work, school, and an infant daughter dividing his attention.

His grandson once told me about a broken shower seat that had contributed to a fall. I showed them how to order a replace- ment, but it didn't happen. My patient had trouble placing a shopping order. How could he be the steward of his complex medical history?

For doctors the boundaries of our obligations can be unclear. Working in a flawed system only amplifies this dilemma. Anything to help a patient, right? My colleagues and I regularly do things outside the scope of medical care simply because a patient needs them. I once rummaged through chutes of dirty laundry trying to find a patient's glasses, which had vanished during his transfer from the emergency room to the hospital ward. (Amazingly, I found them.) In that way, we like to think our work is fundamentally different from other professions. We are guided by a moral compass that is the patient's needs.

People may find it morally repugnant for a doctor to categorize anything that helps a patient as "not my job," but they likely wouldn't react to a lawyer or an accountant saying so. I know this from the reaction to Michael and Leah Champion's story after I first published it as an article. The most common critique I heard questioned why a provider at the nursing home didn't call over. Why didn't the health care workers make more of an effort?

This criticism may feel natural. But ultimately it asks health care workers to dilute our skills into sending faxes. It shifts blame onto individuals instead of focusing on sustainable systemic changes. And it finds a health care system propped up by after-hours clerical work acceptable.

My friend and I are both right. Patients, when they are capable, often *want* to take ownership of their medical stories because it is their future at stake. But some can't. Then what happens? The outcomes mirror deeper societal divides. Without a seamless system, we all suffer, but we don't all suffer equally. Cancer eventually stole a lot from Sarah Leary—her left breast, several lymph nodes, and months of precious time—but it left intact her mind and ability to navigate a complex world. She had the wherewithal to repeatedly call a medical records department and cut through bureaucratic barriers. Then there are those like Michael Champion who have a devoted and savvy family member like his wife, Leah.

What about everyone else?

❖

ALL THAT SAID, everyone who is capable should know a few vital facts of their medical history for one simple reason: it is in their best interest. Medical problems don't follow a script. Something may go wrong when you lack the luxury of complete records: no charts, no flash drives, and no binders. If you're, say, flying on an airplane and a medical emergency happens, what would you want the doctor on the plane to know about you?

A few years ago, on a stiflingly humid day near the end of summer, I was flying home to San Francisco from Houston when a man suddenly collapsed in the aisle. I bolted up from my seat and pushed through a small crowd that was already threatening to block my path to him. "Let me through please, I am a doctor," I called out.

I knelt beside him. He looked to be in his sixties, pale, with a thin gloss of sweat over his forehead. His body lay limp across the aisle. I shook his shoulders and called out: "Sir? Can you hear me?" His eyes fluttered, and he mumbled something. I felt my first flash of relief: this wasn't a true cardiopulmonary arrest, the most serious and deadly of medical emergencies in any situation, much less at thirty thousand feet. I placed two fingers over his carotid artery and confirmed that his pulse was strong.

The flight attendant handed me a medical kit. It was sparse. I pulled out a blood pressure cuff and placed it around his wrist. I retrieved a pulse oximeter and placed it over his index finger. It struck me that this was like running a rapid response in the hospital, a role I had played many times, but with bare-bones equipment and an audience. The latter was especially bizarre. People were leaning into the aisle to watch, mouths agape.

"What happened?" I asked as he came to. "Did you feel dizzy or lightheaded? Has this ever happened before? Are you feeling any chest pressure? Any shortness of breath?" And then the basics: "What are your medical conditions? What medications do you take? Any heart disease? Diabetes?" I was mentally cataloging and triaging the possible culprits of syncope: arrhythmia, hypoglycemia, orthostatic hypotension, vasovagal response, seizure, stroke, pulmonary embolism.

"I didn't feel dizzy, no, just weak. I take metoprolol, Coumadin, aspirin, and Lipitor," he rattled off. "The list is in my wallet." A second wave of relief washed over me. This man knew his medical history. I had something to go on.

"Why do you take Coumadin?" I asked. "Afib," he answered, shorthand for the irregular heart rhythm condition atrial fibrillation. "When was your last dose?" "This morning." Each new piece of information reshuffled the list in my mind. The odds of a pulmonary embolism were small when someone was on active blood thinners. But now I was also concerned about the consequences of a fall while on both Coumadin and aspirin. The aisle was tight, and he went down hard. Did he strike his head?

I used a thin plastic stethoscope to listen to his heart and his lungs, closing my eyes as I tried to tune out the loud background humming of the plane. I counted above ninety beats per minute, on the faster side, but with the regular *lub-dub, lub-dub* rhythm. I performed a focused neurologic exam—hold your hands out straight with your palms facing up, close your eyes, and keep your hands exactly where they were; can you repeat this sentence after me?—and shone my phone light into each pupil, watching it contract.

The story was coming together. This was the third leg of a flight from Europe. He didn't eat or drink much all day. He passed out once before, on a similarly hot day when he had walked a lot and forgotten to drink. All signs on my exam pointed to dehydration.

A flight attendant tapped my shoulder. "Do you need anything else?"

"How long until we're on the ground?" I asked.

She looked at a map, showing us somewhere over Arizona. "About ninety minutes."

I asked her to bring him some orange juice. Then we helped him back to his seat, and I held onto the medical kit. I checked on him several more times until we landed. His blood pressure and oxygen never dipped. His pulse remained regular. When we landed in San Francisco, we were met by two paramedics. I relayed what happened, and they scribbled some notes by hand. I recommended a head CT scan at a local emergency department to rule out a bleed on Coumadin. They thanked me.

As I watched the paramedics help him onto a gurney on the tarmac, I thought about how that man was the poster child of taking ownership over his medical story. By having his medical elevator pitch ready, he handed me tools as valuable as any blood pressure cuff or stethoscope to help him when it mattered most. He was his own advocate, the keeper of his medical narrative, sharing it with a stranger on a plane who he trusted would receive it to help him.

I never learned what happened to him. It was no longer my place.

BACK IN THE CLINIC with Sarah Leary, nearing the end of our visit, we discovered that there was one piece of information missing. There was an old X-ray from before she got cancer, she remembered, showing a bony growth on her hip the radiologist had read as most likely benign. How important was it now?

That thought hung in the air as the usual paths opened before me. I could add tracking it down to a long list of administrative to-dos after my workday ended. I could ask Sarah to retrieve it. Or we could move on. I could offer my recommendations based on a story that was 97 percent complete instead of 100 percent, with a few pages ripped out but the rest mostly intact.

I felt good with the last option. I suggested there was no need to biopsy the bone lesion, which didn't look concerning on her more recent PET scan.

Sarah nodded. The visit was over. I was typing up patient instructions. She was packing up her briefcase of records.

"I don't mean to harp on it," she suddenly said. "But that old X-ray? Would it be helpful to see it yourself?"

I shrugged. "It's not *necessary*," I said. "But sure, if I'm given the choice, complete is always better than incomplete."

We looked at each other. I could see that she was turning this over in her head.

"I'll get it to you," Sarah said. "Just in case."

Chapter 3

Making Computers Work for Us

BEFORE HE HAD REACHED HIS TWENTY-FIFTH BIRTHDAY, A young man I'll call Mitch Garter was hospitalized nearly one hundred times. Blame his kidneys. A healthy kidney pushes electrolytes like potassium and ions like hydrogen out through the urine while absorbing just enough back into the bloodstream to maintain a tight balance at all times. But Mitch was born with an illness that impaired his kidneys from doing these very specific tasks. As a result, he lost excessive amounts of potassium every time he used the bathroom. He spent his life pursuing a nuanced medication regimen to balance his electrolytes in the long term, but in the short term he had to catch up by taking a multitude of potassium pills throughout each day. Any misstep, even sleeping in or eating a mistimed breakfast, could upset the balance quickly and dangerously.

One day as a senior resident admitting patients to the hospital, I received a page from the emergency room about a young man with a critically low potassium reading. As I called back, I clicked open Mitch's electronic chart and pulled up the extraordinarily low number: 1.8 (normal is around 4.0 mmol/L). "You must know him, right?" the emergency doctor asked me. I didn't. But with so many hospitalizations, it seemed only a matter of time before every doctor would come to know Mitch. This was my turn.

I walked to the emergency room and pulled back a curtain to

reveal Mitch lying in a hospital bed. His eyes were clenched shut, his body still. "You must be Mitch," I said. He nodded without opening his eyes. I introduced myself and asked how he felt. "It's like all the other times," he said. He knew his potassium was too low when the muscles in his arms and legs would cramp—painfully. Then they would go limp.

I asked if he could lift his arms now. He couldn't. What about your legs? He furrowed his brow and raised the left one about an inch before it collapsed back onto the mattress.

I checked that Mitch was connected to a continuous heart monitor because the biggest risk of a potassium level being out of normal range is arrhythmia. I printed out an electrocardiogram (ECG), a snapshot of his heart rhythm in time, and circled the extra bumps after each T wave called U waves. The irregular pattern was consistent with a critical absence of potassium and was a precursor to more perilous arrhythmias.

The emergency room doctor told me he had ordered 60 milliequivalents (mEq) of potassium. My immediate plan was to give him another hefty dose right there. Then I would admit him to the hospital, pore through his chart, find the formula that had worked the last ten or so times he was hospitalized, and do something close to that. What subsequent doses should I prescribe and how often? How frequently should we draw blood to stay on track? The chart would tell me.

Mitch Garter was different from Michael Champion and Sarah Leary in one key way: all of his medical care had occurred in the same place. This would not be a story of collating records from different hospitals. I didn't have to chase down long-lost potassium dosages that disappeared in fax machines. Everything I could possibly need I had in an electronic file in front of me. Figuring out how to treat the hundred-and-first episode of the same problem seemed as close to following a cookbook as it could get.

SOME DOCTORS MIGHT PROTEST that there's nothing "cookbook" about what we do. None of us powered through a decade or more of intensive medical training—working eighty-hour weeks and overseeing the care of thousands of diverse patients—only to follow a recipe. The beauty of medicine is in its art. We diagnose and treat individuals, not patterns, engaging in complex problem-solving that factors in the distinctive features and oddities of each case.

Although this is one of the great joys of being a doctor, a lot of the practice of medicine also involves recognizing patterns and following blueprints that are known to work. We don't reinvent the wheel with every case of community-acquired pneumonia or congestive heart failure. Diagnostic and treatment plans that have already been worked out tell us how many days of antibiotics are best to eradicate pneumonia or what medications synergize most to preserve cardiac function and prevent heart failure flares. Leaning on past knowledge is also a good start on an individual patient level. Whether I'm treating nausea induced by chemotherapy, choosing an antidepressant to help a patient through a difficult time, or restoring a critically low potassium level caused by a rare congenital kidney disease, one of the most informative questions I can ask patients (and their charts) is, "What has worked for you before?"

These pattern-based parts of medicine are the perfect place for technology to step in, and it's worth pausing to acknowledge how good we have it. The computerized charts we use as doctors are not merely electronic filing cabinets. In addition to storing data, they also embed certain tools to help make sense of that information. When I admit a patient to the hospital with a suspected emphysema flare, for example, I can pull up a set of orders. Rather than remembering and constructing orders from scratch, I run through suggestions typically written for the condition: oxygen through a nasal cannula, nebulized inhalers, prednisone, azithromycin, and even a nicotine patch. If I try to order Haldol for an agitated patient and he's on another medication that could negatively interact with it, the chart alerts me to a potential error. When I want to look at a patient's potassium level, I can visually display in a graph what his numbers within the system have been over time.

But for all the ways today's computerized charts can connect patient data, there's a catch: much of the time, they don't. Somehow, even within one electronic system, the charts have managed to link some data while fracturing other parts of a patient's story even more. Bloat without organization makes it harder to find the information we really need. Roundabout data entry forces health care workers to distract ourselves with hours of extraneous computerized tasks. The result is that we spend exorbitant energy digging for a full story and tidying it for the next doctor, and we still miss things. Digital health expert Mark Savage described the problem with an analogy: "Imagine going to a car rental place and looking for the gas pedal—maybe this time, it's in the backseat."

Griping about too much information after chronicling all the problems of having too little may seem strange. But the problem is not having too many records; the problem is lack of organization. Exchanging information is the first step, but if that information isn't usable, an excess of messy data can fragment a patient's story as much as not having it in the first place.

Unfortunately, this is the current state of affairs: even within a single electronic medical records system, disorganization has fragmented patient stories into a muddled maze of clicks. The electronic charts hold the potential to consolidate data into narratives and augment doctors' decision-making in astonishing ways. Or they can insert detours and bury critical information to slow us down and incubate mistakes. This is one of the great puzzles medicine is grappling with today: How can we realize the full potential of automation? What should this look like, and how do we get there?

Back in the emergency room with Mitch, I had no answer. That is why, as I sat before multibillion-dollar software trying to decipher his case, what I pulled out next was a piece of paper and a pen.

Replacing potassium is one of the first things a doctor learns to do. It's an uninspiring task, usually relegated to first-year residents. As an intern I received literally hundreds of pages from nurses after the morning lab results came back asking me to "please replete." The formula is simple: giving 10 mEq of potassium raises the blood level by approximately 0.1 mmol/L. So if the morning labs came back at 3.8 and your goal is 4.0, you'd give 20 mEq. Replacing potassium is the doctors' equivalent of replacing an empty roll of toilet paper—mindless but someone has got to do it.

That's because as lackluster as this task is, it's also crucial. Potassium is an exquisitely regulated electrolyte. Our kidneys, gut, and brain all play roles in keeping it within a tight range, with any deviation causing harmful effects. In skeletal muscle, low potassium can cause extreme weakness or even paralysis. In heart muscle, a potassium level out of range can lead to arrhythmias and even sudden cardiac death.

When someone's potassium is out of whack, other imbalances can happen. Magnesium deficiency can occur simultaneously and aggravate treatment attempts to get potassium back to normal. Abnormal amounts of acid in the bloodstream can cause potassium to shift into and out of cells, further disturbing the levels in the blood. It's essential to sort out cause from effect, and the order of repairing different problems matters.

Mitch's case added another complication. I looked at his electronic chart tab listing the potassium doses he took at home and briefly thought a zero had been added by mistake. His daily doses were multiple times higher than anything I was accustomed to prescribing.

Then I clicked on the "Notes" tab in Mitch's chart. I clicked a few more buttons to filter them by hospital discharge summaries. As I read through prior doctors' accounts of Mitch's medical care, I was struck by the inconsistencies. Sometimes his potassium was replaced smoothly over one to two days, and he was discharged shortly thereafter. Other times his potassium yo-yoed, requiring ICU transfers and extra medications to get it back down. Every medical team seemed to create its own plan and gave different doses and rates of infusion, making it easy to overshoot or under-shoot. There didn't seem to be a formula for something I thought would have been formulaic by now.

I decided I'd try the approach I used with Sarah Leary. Maybe I would be lucky, and Mitch would have the magic formula at the tip of his tongue. I braced myself for the retort, "Didn't you *read* my chart?" But the most important thing was getting his care right. If he had answers, I'd welcome them.

I went back to his bedside. "I was reading your chart," I said, "and noticed some different ways your other doctors have treated you when this happens. What helps you most when you're in the hospital?"

"Potassium," Mitch said. I pressed for more details, but he couldn't tell me anything. He, like many patients, deferred to his trusted doctors on the details. Why shouldn't he?

I went back to my paper and pen. The typical repletion for-mula—10 mEq adds approximately 0.1 mmol/L to a blood level—meant that to get his potassium from 1.8 to a normal level of at least 3.5, he needed at least 170 mEq. He had already received 60 mEq from the emergency room doctor. That left 110 mEq.

It was straightforward math, but as I typed an order into his chart, I balked: 100 mEq is literally the dose of potassium used in lethal injection. The chart responded by trying to correct me. That's a much higher dose than usual, it prompted. Are you sure?

ASK ANY DOCTOR how they approach the chart-scouring part of a new medical case, and you'll get a different answer. When I sign into a patient's electronic chart, I am greeted with choices. Lining the top of my screen are three rows of up to a dozen tabs each. I can choose to look at encounters (for example, office visits and telephone calls), provider notes, procedures, labs, radiology reports, medications, referrals, media (outside scans), and a few more. Along the left of my screen are over a dozen more choices— a patient's vital signs, recent height and weight, medications and allergies (again), recent visits (also again), insurance information, vaccinations, and more. Once I click on anything, the choices multiply like Russian dolls. If I click on notes, for instance, I can filter by author or type of visit. If I look at results, I can choose which lab results I want to see and how I want them displayed.

My own approach has differed depending on my role. When admitting patients to the hospital, I always went for discharge summaries first. As an oncology consulting physician, I usually looked at the pathology tab before anything else. When I'm seeing new patients in the clinic, my first click to orient myself is the medication list.

What each of these situations share, however, is that there's too much information to read everything. That fact may surprise some people. But big data is *big*. The widely used electronic chart system Epic is so complex that the company has designated some providers as "Super Users," who are tasked with teaching chart tricks to others. To put it in numbers, the electronic chart for a patient like Mitch runs to tens of thousands of words. Parts of the chart are searchable; other parts are not. Some data are where you'd expect them, while others are not. Many parts are repetitive. Other parts are irrelevant. The electronic charts have built the haystack, but they haven't yet evolved to find the needle. As I click around, searching for what I need, I think of the words of Samuel Taylor Coleridge: "Water, water everywhere, nor any drop to drink."

And consider the other relevant numbers. While I was treating Mitch, I was responsible for fourteen other hospitalized patients. I was getting paged five to ten times an hour. I had thirty minutes to respond to the emergency room about each new patient they wished to admit.

That doesn't leave much time to dig, yet that's what we have to do. As a new doctor, I once accepted a patient transfer to the hospital wards after he had spent two weeks in the cardiac care unit (CCU). He had intermittent episodes of ventricular tachycardia, a serious arrhythmia, and was started on a medication called amiodarone to treat it. This medication works best when administered at high doses over several days to reach a cumulative dose, after which it's tapered to a maintenance dose. I remember asking another doctor where in the chart I could see how much amiodarone my patient had already received. I was surprised by the answer: no place. I had to click through records of the patient's different days in the CCU, pinpoint every time a dose was charted, and then add them up myself. It was like signing into your online banking account to find each check deposited in a separate tab, which you have to track down and add manually to see your total. The method was labor intensive and error prone.

The disorganization is not just in retrieving data but inputting that information. Every time I order something as simple as an ultrasound, I am greeted with a slew of choices that could lead me inadvertently to pick the wrong one. Every time I do a procedure as routine as a Pap smear, I wade through clicks. I answer myriad questions: What is the collection date? When was the patient's last menses? What is the specimen type? What is the specimen source? Is the test for screening or diagnosis? If I try to sign my order before answering these questions, the computer blocks me.

While all of this data can ultimately help us understand important medical trends, the input process on an everyday basis is onerous, tedious, and clerical. The same alerts that have the power to notify us of important findings also bombard us, leaving no choice but to click through sometimes just to get by. It feels like receiving dozens of spam emails from which you cannot unsubscribe.

Then there's redundancy. I once tried to explain to some engineer friends how I made my rounds of hospitalized patients every morning. My explanation horrified everyone. I print out a document from the electronic chart with the morning's vital signs, test results, and medication list. Then I scour the chart for other things I want to know about my patients, such as specialist recommendations and events from overnight, and scribble them in by hand. After I see all the patients, I type my handwritten scribbles *back* into the computer into a daily progress note.

One study published in 2021 examined nearly three million medical notes input into the charts over a decade. The proportion of text identical to the previous note increased over that time— from 48 percent to 59 percent. A patient's chart might be cluttered with the fact that she smokes cigarettes and is at risk for lung cancer, but when ordering a lung cancer CT screen of her chest, I am prompted to answer reasons why and must type it in again. When I write a note, instead of importing test results directly from one part of the chart to another, I pull up separate tabs, highlight, copy, close the tabs, and paste.

Many researchers have now studied the experiences I and so many other doctors live, and the data are stunning even to me. These things add up. A paper in 2018 found that ordering Tylenol required anywhere between fourteen and sixty-two clicks—with the confusion causing errors in up to 30 percent of cases. The number of clicks made in one ten-hour shift in the emergency room can approach four thousand.

This doesn't jibe with how human cognition works. Many times I've been more grateful for one well-written paragraph from another doctor than for any number of tabs containing disparate pieces of data. It's time consuming and exhausting—not to mention susceptible to errors—to re-create the narrative myself.

Researchers are finding clever ways to capture data about the damage. In one study, researchers asked twenty-five ICU doctors to wear glasses that tracked the size of their pupils. (Pupil size is known to shrink with fatigue.) The doctors then worked with electronic charts. They reviewed four patient cases, after which the researchers quizzed them. The researchers found that, based on their pupil size, all the doctors experienced fatigue at least once. Eighty percent felt fatigue within the first twenty-two minutes of interacting with the charts. Studies like these validate my fears—that my brainpower is being depleted by clicks when I need it to do the work of being a doctor.

None of these problems make sense. From an engineering perspective, we have the capabilities to tackle any one of the electronic charts' issues. With all of a patient's data in one place, the possibilities to put the pieces together automatically and improve patient care are endless. So why have the charts garbled that data into a fragmented mess instead?

PART OF THE ANSWER lies not in technology but in the unintended consequences of an initial design. When the great shift from paper charts to electronic ones began, the government wanted to stimulate the entire country to go paperless. They believed in standardization (correctly, I should add—who wants the gas pedal in the backseat?). In order to track which hospitals were adopting the technology, the Centers for Medicare and Medicaid Services, the federal agency behind the operation, set standards known as "Meaningful Use," where a slew of metrics had to be met electronically for hospitals to receive funding.

But because these metrics were fundamentally designed for billing, not for patient care, doctors were required to jump through all sorts of clunky hoops to prove their clinics were worthy of reimbursement. For example, health care workers had to document in very specific ways items like a patient's smoking status and family medical history, whether those patients were being seen for a cold or end-of-life care. With these factors irrelevant at best and distracting at worst to the medical situation at hand, doctors' use of copy-paste ran rampant so they could get through their workdays. The electronic ecosystem became littered with useless information, while important things got buried. Over time we have just kept adding to the garbage pile. (Many doctors now pejoratively dub "Meaningful Use" as "Meaningless Abuse.")

The result today is that the same technology that possesses so much power to simplify labor has drastically increased it. A poll by Stanford Medicine researchers of more than five hundred primary care doctors found that 63 percent believe electronic health records have generally improved care. However, 71 percent felt that electronic charts contribute to physician burnout; 49 percent felt the charts detracted from their medical effectiveness; and 59 percent believed they need a complete overhaul. And everyone notices: doctors and patients alike lament the loss of eye contact as technology comes between them.

In perhaps the greatest ironic twist, our current solution for these computer glitches is employing more human labor. Scribes stand in the corner of our exam rooms, transcribing our words into laptops as we dictate aloud. Medical assistants clean up medication lists and hand us notes they've printed out before we knock on patients' clinic room doors. Nurse practitioners and physician assistants enter orders and save them into the computer, diving through the dozens of requisite clicks so that doctors can simply click to sign. We hire people to serve the needs of the electronic charts. It was supposed to be the other way around.

I OVERRODE THE CHART'S WARNING and signed for 100 mEq of potassium to be given, but in liquid solution form. Next I started a continuous potassium drip at 20 mEq per hour, infused through his port. We drew blood one hour later, and I was pleased by the number: 2.8. We were making progress but not overshooting.

We continued to draw blood every two hours. By the evening his potassium was 3.4, so we spaced out his blood draws to every four hours and slowed the drip. The next morning we transitioned Mitch back to his home regimen. We ordered medications for nausea that he could take if needed. We watched the U waves on his ECG flatten and vanish. Mitch began to wiggle his fingers and toes, then lift his arms and legs. His other metabolic disturbances, including the acid levels in his blood, normalized.

It was only then, when we were preparing to discharge Mitch, that I found it. Under a tab labeled "problem list" was the magic formula I had been seeking. It was a few short sentences written by his regular nephrologist, explaining what doses of potassium to give, by what route, and how often. Then, in all caps, was a warning: DO NOT GIVE BICARB EVEN IF THERE IS ACIDOSIS, AS THAT WILL LOWER THE POTASSIUM.

My mind reeled. My first feeling was pride; the potassium replenishment plan we constructed from scratch was nearly identical to the ideal recipe. Then came relief. We had come to the same conclusion to avoid bicarb, a medication we often give to reverse acidosis. However, the decision wasn't a straightforward one. After the thought initially crossed my mind, we worked through the pros and cons of doing so. I wondered if other doctors had missed the expert's instructions just as I had.

Mitch always did fine. But suppose I had given bicarb and Mitch's potassium dropped so low that he required ICU care. Suppose, heaven forbid, even worse—the potassium bottomed out to the point that his heart stopped beating, a code was called, and a team descended to pound on his chest and shock him back to life. Who would be responsible? Me—the doctor who didn't read the chart carefully enough to avoid giving an ampule of bicarb—or the electronic chart, which should have helped me see the information that mattered most? I imagined a malpractice lawyer sitting in a quiet room, sans pager, taking the weeks required to read Mitch's chart thoroughly. The lawyer could point out the information was all here; the doctor just didn't follow it.

Like most doctors, I know the statistics: the odds of facing a malpractice lawsuit in a long medical career are about 50 percent. I know that if I make an error, I should be upfront about what happened and apologize. I learned this not only because it is the right thing to do but also because it makes doctors less likely to be sued.

I also know that an error can stem from the electronic chart's flaws, and at the end of the day, I am still accountable. While the electronic charts have reduced some errors that lead to lawsuits, they've frighteningly increased others. A paper published in 2019 examined 248 malpractice cases from 2012 to 2013 in which the charts were implicated. While these constituted less than 1 percent of total malpractice cases, many claims were related to fragmented data—even within one system.

One claim involved test results that were recorded in multiple locations in the chart. Because of this dispersion of data, the medical team failed to pick up on a downward trajectory of concerning vital signs and lab tests. The patient died of sepsis. Another claim showed a positive test result for cervical cancer entered into the problem list (eerily, the same place Mitch's instructions from his nephrologist were located); the doctor, expecting to find it in the test results section, did not discover it until the patient's visit a year later. Yet another found a critical ultrasound result routed to the wrong tab; this doctor, too, didn't see the result until a year later, delaying a diagnosis of cancer.

Another study, published in 2013, reported that over half of primary care doctors believe the electronic charts make it easy to miss results—with a whopping 30 percent reporting that they personally had missed abnormal findings. Of note, the doctors often attributed their mistakes to noise—too much information—compared to vanished data, with the doctors who reported receiving too many alerts more likely to recount missing important findings.

These stories were terrifying in their familiarity. And what are our solutions? We've gotten so desperate for ways to signal "important" in the chart it's almost comical: we bold, we turn the font red, we blow up its size, we underline, we use all caps, we pepper the text with exclamation points. We also use our own makeshift organizational systems outside the charts. My white coat pockets bulge with scrap paper and four-color pens. I have separate follow-up lists, master lists of to-dos outside the charts. It doesn't matter what your system is. But you need something.

I thought about this as I wrote a discharge summary for Mitch. I paused, pondering the best place to pass off my newfound discovery of the tried-and-true formula. I recognized the irony: by writing more in the chart, I was by definition making it longer, more convoluted, and more repetitive. At the same time, I needed to give the next doctor the best chance of finding what she or he needed. Realistically, whenever I need to pass along critical information, I go around the chart. In the age of multibillion-dollar software and big data, the safest course of action is to email or call my colleagues directly. Sometimes I leave notes at their desks. But in this case, I didn't know who the next doctor treating Mitch would be. There was no phone call I could make, no destination for a nomadic, urgent post-it note.

NOT ALL HOPE IS LOST. As the failed potential of the charts is being realized, doctors and others are working furiously to rectify the situation—and they're drawing lessons from other initiatives that have improved patient safety.

I learned about the process to improve systems, known as quality improvement, when I volunteered to lead a task force to improve an issue near and dear to my heart: fragmented communication between the emergency room and the hospital wards. The only problem was that I had no idea how to lead such a task force. I asked a colleague who had successfully carried out quality-improvement projects to help, and I sat in his windowless office one afternoon as he drew with a marker on a whiteboard. There I learned a new language. I learned the language of something called PDSA—plan, do, study, act. I learned how to ask myself "five whys" to home in on the root cause of a problem.

He told me a story about these tools in practice. At his previous workplace, one doctor identified a problem: doctors in the emergency room were not doing bedside echocardiograms for medical issues that typically warranted them. So a small group of doctors did a deep dive into barriers. "Why?" they asked themselves. And then when one barrier was identified, they asked again: "Why?" It wasn't lack of training. It wasn't lack of time. The root cause, it turns out, was that the emergency room doctors couldn't find the ultrasound machine. As ridiculous as this sounds, I nodded along because I had faced the same problem. I thought back to the nights I spent wandering—up to the ICU, down to the emergency department, circling the wards—trying to track down a precious bedside ultrasound machine. Doctors (myself included) would borrow them and then either forget or not know where to return them.

How did the group solve that problem? They designated a spot for the machine and used bright yellow duct tape to construct a square on the floor. From then on, that was the ultrasound's home. I had to smile. With all of our medical knowledge and training, the grand solution was taping the floor. But it worked. It was successful because the group identified one problem, interviewed the right people to understand it, and crafted a solution that addressed the root cause. They didn't go too big or try to reinvent.

I kept this in mind when I met with my own team of about ten physicians. One of the problems we identified was that doctors rushed to admit patients to the hospital before all the lab or scan results had come back. Sometimes, for example, a patient was transferred to the medical floors only to have a scan result return suggesting the problem was actually surgical. "Why does this happen?" I asked. Someone brought up the three-hour limit. At our hospital we aim to make a discharge decision—send home or admit—for every patient in the emergency room after three hours. "Why does the three-hour limit exist?" I asked. "Another QI [quality improvement] project," someone quipped.

At that moment, I had a new understanding of why fixing anything in our electronic charts was so difficult: trying to solve one problem created another. Our electronic charts have congealed over time into the product we have now. Trying to chip away at any one defect can cause other structures to crumble.

I learned a lot over those few weeks. The guiding principle is slow, incremental change. Resist quick fixes with unintended consequences. Monitor outcomes, incorporate feedback, and tweak the plan in real time. Involve all stakeholders. If you're improving communication between the emergency department and the hospital wards, for example, you have to talk to both teams of doctors. You also have to talk to the emergency department clerk, the charge nurses, and the information technology team.

How can we apply this logic to the electronic charts? It seems obvious, but a good technological solution makes things easier. I sat in on enough unsuccessful project solutions to see a theme. To patch a hole, someone would suggest adding something: incorporate another checklist, click some more boxes, fire off more intrusive alerts. But this led to more manual tasks that extracted time and mental energy from doctors. Going back to Mark Savage's imaginary rental car problem, it would be like taping a memo to the windshield of each faulty car: brake on the left, gas pedal in the backseat. The best solutions simplify.

I talked to many who tried simplifying the process, with varying levels of success. An internist at the University of Utah named Devin Horton shared one of the more optimistic stories. As a new faculty member, Horton noticed that patients with sepsis were not always receiving appropriate treatment with antibiotics right away. The signs that sepsis could be brewing—such as a fever, a fast heart rate, and low blood pressure—were all in the electronic charts, but they either weren't being looked at or weren't interpreted correctly. It reminded me of the instructions from Mitch's nephrologist: how could the chart better inform us of what mattered? Around the same time Horton was noticing this, he went to a conference and attended a talk on recognizing sepsis that ended with a call to action. Inspired, he drafted a plan on the plane ride home. "I was bright-eyed and ambitious," he told me.

From there he followed all the rules of engagement I'd come to learn distinguish a successful project. He started with a pilot program. He held meetings and involved stakeholders from the get-go. He and colleagues used the vital signs in the chart to generate a score that quantified how sick the patient was. When the score reached a certain number, the chart automatically alerted the charge nurse and primary medical team. If it reached an even higher level, it alerted the rapid response medical team and the ICU. Nurses had leeway to draw baseline sepsis lab samples, such as blood cultures and lactic acid tests. When the doctor arrived, a sepsis order set populated the chart to let her order additional treatments and tests.

With every step, Horton listened to feedback and made changes in real time, adjusting thresholds to alert providers without overwhelming them. "We wanted to know who was getting sick, not get dinged about every person in the hospital," he said. While the hoped-for decrease in mortality ultimately didn't appear, they did find a reduction in a patient's length of stay in the hospital and lowered costs.

When I asked what he learned, Horton acknowledged the power of simplifying. Effective solutions don't add work but lean on what the technology is already doing. "Providers have a lot of stuff on their plates; you have to be careful when you put something else on," he said. "I get that now."

FOR ALL THIS TO WORK, we must remember who's in charge. The ideal division of labor between technology and doctors is like a self-driving car—effective for offloading the basic tasks but still requiring a driver who can take over and hit the emergency brake. A doctor must retain autonomy to override the automation—at any time, for any reason.

Another example comes from my time working night shifts during residency, when I was responsible for managing dozens of patients dispersed throughout the hospital. My work during these shifts was mostly reactive; I wasn't mapping out who needed long-term care facilities but keeping everyone alive until the morning. Every evening I received a printed sign-out from the daytime doctors, and I circled the sickest patients in red. These were the ones I would check on throughout the night. For everyone else, I waited to hear about a problem.

A few hours into my shift one night, a problem cropped up: a bedside nurse paged me about a forty-four-year-old woman who had a bloody bowel movement. "Do you want to see it?" the nurse asked. I briefly clicked through the patient's chart and gathered a complicated medical history of an autoimmune disorder that was now affecting her gut in ways no one fully understood. I also flipped through my paper sign-out as I walked to the patient's room, which was two floors up and all the way on the other side of the hospital. This wasn't someone I had circled. "Stable," my one-liner said. My printed notes also told me that she had an endoscopy and colonoscopy earlier that day to take biopsies of suspicious-looking areas. Some residual bleeding after the procedure wouldn't be unusual, I thought.

But when I got to the room, I saw that it was more than just a residual ooze. Drops on the floor were the bright red breadcrumbs leading to the commode, where the nurse had saved the stool as promised. But the patient's vital signs were perfectly normal, and she looked well, calmly jabbing a plastic spoon into a pudding cup when I arrived. I asked how she felt. "A little dizzy when I stood up but better now," she said. Her labs from that afternoon showed that her hemoglobin levels were stable and far above the threshold where I would consider a blood transfusion.

I made sure her blood type was up to date and ordered a complete blood count and coagulation lab tests, one liter of normal saline to infuse now, and two units of blood to have on standby. I asked the nurse to replace her IV with a larger bore, at least 16- or 18-gauge, and to place a second one in the other arm. I looked through her medication list for any blood thinners and canceled the aspirin that was scheduled to restart the next morning. Finally, I talked to the charge nurse about moving the patient to a bed closer to my workroom.

With all of that set in motion, I did other work. I triaged calls from the emergency room, admitted a new patient, did rounds on my sickest patients, and fielded pages about everyone else. It was the normal work of a busy night shift.

About an hour later, I returned to a computer to check on the results from the woman upstairs. The chart got my attention with an alert: the patient was now flagged as septic. Her heart rate was high, her breathing was fast, and her blood pressure was low. Similar to the University of Utah, we had our own sepsis alert system. As if on cue, my pager blared: RAPID RESPONSE. I ran to the patient's new room, fortunately now only a hallway away from me, and was met by a rapid response nurse who had also been summoned by the chart. By the time I arrived, a full set of vital signs had been taken, and blood work had been drawn. Alert, standardize, delegate—so far so good.

I looked at the monitor and saw a heart rate in the 140s and a blood pressure of 84 over 50. The patient, who an hour earlier was eating chocolate pudding and telling me she was fine, was now sweaty and mumbling incoherently. She turned in bed, revealing a pool of fresh blood.

"Run a second liter of normal saline, wide open," I said to the bedside nurse. "What do we have for access?"

"Left antecubital IV, 20-gauge."

"Just one?" I asked, also noting that it hadn't been upgraded to the larger size. "What about the second one?"

She looked at me. She was a different bedside nurse from the one I had asked to place the IV an hour before. I realized what had happened: when the patient transferred rooms as I had requested, the instructions to place a second IV fell to the bottom of the to-do list if it was even passed on at all. I felt a flash of panic. What else hadn't been done?

"Do we have a complete blood count and coagulation labs?" I asked. "And two units of blood on standby?"

The blood work I had ordered was thankfully done. But while the order for two units of blood was signed into the computer, the actual blood products were nowhere to be seen.

I asked the nurse standing next to the portable computer to read me the results. She scrolled for a moment and then read the dismal numbers aloud. The picture was coming into focus. The patient's blood was not able to clot the way it should, and after a procedure earlier in the day snipped her intestines for the biopsies, her gut couldn't heal. So she bled.

"Doc, do you want to start antibiotics?" the rapid response nurse asked me then. "For the sepsis?"

"No," I answered. "This isn't septic shock. It's hemorrhagic shock."

She looked unsure. "How do you know it's a hemorrhage?"

It was like looking at a chair and being asked, "But how do you know it's a chair?"

I explained that the bleed mimicked the signs of sepsis, and our biggest priority right now was to transfuse blood. I didn't want to waste our one IV on antibiotics the patient did not need. I asked the rapid response nurse to call the blood bank and ask for a massive transfusion pack; this would get us more than the two units of packed red blood cells I ordered earlier, including platelets and fresh frozen plasma to help her blood clot. I requested a dose of vitamin K be given immediately, also to help with clotting. Then I dialed the ICU fellow with one hand while I again took the patient's blood pressure with the other: now it was 75 over 45. Her heart rate had jumped to the 160s. "Ms. C," I called out her name. "Can you tell me where you are?"

"I don't feel good," she responded.

A second rapid response nurse came up behind the first and murmured to her. Then he turned to me: "Are you sure you don't want to start vancomycin, Doc? Or Zosyn?" He was naming antibiotics.

The patient needed blood, she needed it fast, and we had limited routes to get it in. A nurse was working on placing an IV in her right hand while another worked on her foot. Meanwhile, everyone was asking me about antibiotics for the "sepsis" about which the chart alerted them. The room had filled with well-meaning and highly trained providers, all of whom, I realized, could blindly follow an electronic algorithm while the patient hemorrhaged in front of our eyes.

"I can't breathe," she announced then. Her oxygen level fell from 97 percent to 80 percent, and I gave the OK to the respiratory therapist who immediately began to bag-mask her. He placed the plastic covering over her mouth and nose and squeezed the attached balloon, pushing oxygen into her lungs. "Ms. C, can you hear me?" She was slurring her words. I checked her blood pressure again, and it was 60 over 40. The fluids were still running through her single IV.

Just as I called for a syringe of a vasopressor medication to have in hand in order to revive her blood pressure, the rapid response nurse announced, "Second IV in!" She secured tape around the IV in the patient's right hand. A different nurse appeared, panting and triumphant, and delivered a cooler of blood products. We connected one unit of red blood cells to an IV in one arm and a unit of fresh frozen plasma to the IV in the other. Over the next hour, I carefully directed what went in each IV as we gave the patient multiple units of blood products. Her blood pressure drifted up. Her oxygen returned to 95 percent. She became coherent again. "What's going on?" she asked. "You had a bleed," I said, "but we are taking care of you."

Over the next few hours, we transferred her to the ICU where she stabilized. The gastroenterologist came in and performed a bedside colonoscopy under the close watch of beeping ICU monitors. The culprit—a bleeding spot of large intestine—was zapped with heat until the bleeding stopped. By the next morning, the patient was transferred back to the wards, and two days later she was home.

She was OK. But it was close—too close. Medicine is all about anticipating complications and preparing for them two steps before they strike. Scrambling is a surefire path to disaster. I kept thinking about it later. I asked myself the "five whys." At first I shook my fist against electronic algorithms. By asking for the transfer to a bed closer to me, for example, I had sent the patient onto a conveyor belt of clicks, checklists, and documentation. Compared to the electronic gymnastics required to complete the transfer, upgrading an IV and placing a second one—both verbal orders given right before the patient was moved—were easy to let slip. It culminated in the bleeding versus sepsis conundrum. The chart told me it was sepsis, and so at first glance other health care providers believed it was sepsis. "Are you sure you don't want to start vancomycin?" they all asked.

Later, in a quiet room and out of my blood-stained clogs, I examined the data on sepsis in our hospital. In a world where the problem is too often failing to follow guidelines that work, the protocol was implemented for good reason. The alerts correctly identified sepsis in many cases and led to earlier administration of antibiotics in the sickest patients who needed them. As I thought more about it, I realized the technology, imperfect as it was, had worked as intended. The alert got me, two critical care nurses, a pharmacist, and a respiratory therapist to the bedside urgently and without delay. It alerted us to catastrophe, even if it got the details wrong on what kind of catastrophe it was. The recommendation to start antibiotics was just that—a suggestion, not a dictate or hard stop. At that point, a human stepped in and overrode the technology, providing care to the patient based on the reality on the ground.

I mentioned this story to Devin Horton. To two doctors, it was obvious that lots of things besides sepsis can cause low blood pressure, a fast heart rate, and rapid breathing. We can debate the exact thresholds that should trigger a sepsis alert until we're blue in the face. But

I agreed with what Horton said next: "All of those situations require someone to see the patient and think about doing something."

MEDICINE TAKES COURAGE. It takes courage to run up to a hemorrhaging patient and command a room. But medicine has also demanded courage from me in less flashy ways. It takes courage to put your ego aside and check what has worked before—just to be safe—no matter how many times you have done something. It takes courage to say, "Let me dig some more, and I'll get back to you," in a culture that values immediate decisions as a sign of wisdom. Often it takes the most courage not to plow ahead but to pause. That pause can come from anyone: from patients, family members, and other care providers who challenge one another to think a bit harder, buck hierarchies, and raise questions.

This courage has an end point, and it's to care for one another in a way that is fully human. Cumbersome charts erode the human element in care in ways that cannot be measured as easily as faulty medication doses. When sitting down years later to write Mitch's story, I had forgotten some details of his case, but one thing stayed with me. It was the look on his face that first day when I went back to his bedside and asked what treatment worked best for him. His expression was not confusion. It was not frustration. It was something deeper, a kind of despair I didn't fully understand. I realized I had no idea what Mitch's life was like—choking down many potassium pills a day, tethered to the next 911 call that would bring him to the hospital.

I like to imagine a world where I paused. Maybe we would talk. Maybe we would be silent. Maybe he would share, and I would listen. Maybe I would find out why he hadn't taken his potassium that morning. Maybe I'd have words of advice or comfort. Maybe he'd consider them.

But there, then, I did none of these things. Instead, I went back to my computer and made eye contact with the pixels. I have regret about this moment, but it is not the regret of making the wrong choice. There is no world in which it would have been correct to sit and hold Mitch's hand while his potassium slowly drifted downward and induced a fatal arrhythmia. What I regret is that I was forced into this choice by a system that extracts inordinate amounts of time, energy, and neuroticism just to take care of the basics. If we don't prioritize change, that system will burn us out. It already is doing so. Our relationships with electronic charts reroute limited resources of cognition and caring to clicking boxes. We will have less and less left to spend on what matters most.

Yet I remain hopeful. We have now identified three lampposts for truly meaningful use of data in health care: 1) share it among doctors; 2) give patients access; 3) organize it. In the early 2000s, Mitch's story would have been passed to me through indecipherable handwriting on loose-leaf paper. We have knocked things down, rebuilt, and moved forward. Our charts are our stories: living records of our medical past, present, and future. We must recognize the urgency in getting this part right.

I did see Mitch once more. A few months later, I was on rotation in my hospital's nephrology clinic and happened to see his name on the day's schedule. I knocked on the door and reintroduced myself. In those thirty minutes, I made a conscious decision not to pull up a computer. I learned about his nausea. I learned that it's easy to skip a potassium pill or two or three when you are trying to hold down a job and your breakfast simultaneously. In that space, I got to know him just a little better. I felt a hint of a connection that was squandered before because I was busy doing the work of a computer and for a computer. That work kept me occupied, and it kept me from being present. I don't pretend to know Mitch, not on any deep level. But it was a start.

Part 2

Lost to
Follow-Up

Chapter 4

Are You My Doctor?

BY THE NUMBERS, A MAN I'LL CALL JIN WONG, A SIXTY-year-old from China, was in good hands. He had two children, three grandchildren—and thirty-one doctors.

It was a warm September day when he landed at the San Francisco airport, anticipating a month-long stay with his daughter, Vanessa. His plans were unassuming. He would eat good food, play with the grandchildren, and watch his soaps in the living room recliner. But when Vanessa picked him up from the airport, she immediately knew something was wrong. Jin had to stop to catch his breath several times on the short walk to the airport parking lot. That evening, as he bit into the welcome dinner Vanessa had prepared for him, his gums bled.

Vanessa convinced him the soaps would have to wait. They got back in the car and drove to the emergency room.

I was the hematology and oncology fellow covering our hospital's inpatient leukemia ward when I got a page about Jin. I looked at the blood test results from the emergency room and saw that his white blood cell count was sky-high while his platelets and red blood cells were vanishingly low. I pulled his blood smear from the lab and examined it under a microscope. Large, disfigured cells with irregular borders covered the slide. These were leukemia cells called blasts.

I met Jin and Vanessa in the emergency room with a Cantonese medical interpreter at my side. I introduced myself as the oncology doctor. Jin calmly stood up to greet me, while Vanessa's face crumpled and she began to cry. "The emergency doctor said my dad might have leukemia. Is it true?"

As an oncologist, you quickly learn that your presence speaks volumes and that a hard conversation may have begun as soon as you signal who you are. Jin Wong would pass away from his disease. Over the next few months, I tried to answer Vanessa and Jin's questions honestly. I took extra steps to remain by his side through the harrowing journey that is not just serious illness but serious illness with blunted access to health care: Jin did not have U.S. health insurance.

Thus began a different kind of odyssey through a fragmented health care system. How we do (or don't) keep medical data is one way a patient's story is glued together. Another is how we do (or don't) maintain the relationship between a patient and a doctor. Most people have encountered the ways health insurance companies fragment this dynamic by inserting third parties that question doctors' decision-making and expose patients to a post-hoc game of financial risk. It never stops feeling strange for me to counsel patients through the facts: no, I don't know how much this will cost you; your insurance will decide what they will cover after the fact; so do you want the MRI?

Then there's being uninsured. In that situation a patchwork of measures exists to catch patients from falling through completely. But when you get into the particulars of what this patchwork can do, you see a larger judgment about what is considered nonnegotiable, life-saving care. By our nation's standards, at the bottom of the list is the doctor-patient relationship.

The problem is that the doctor-patient relationship is not merely a nice thing to have; it's the crux of effective medicine. Jin Wong would spend the remainder of his life ferrying between doctors, looking for the one who knew his whole story and could lead his care. As much as I wanted to be that doctor for him, I couldn't. I think now of the earnestness of our first meeting—a patient speaking with his doctor—and how easily the relationship would fall apart.

FROM THE MOMENT I MET JIN, I was thinking ahead—way ahead. While my patients catch their breath about the coming hours and days, I am often thinking in years. When moving from the world of the healthy to that of the chronically ill, a person crosses an invisible threshold into a new life: of monitoring, checkups, tinkering, changing course, recalibrating expectations, preventing complications, and living in uncertainty. He becomes tied to health care in a way that is easy to underestimate until one has lived it.

Jin's diagnosis, acute myeloid leukemia, encapsulates this shift. His disease could potentially be cured, but it would require a tough initial chemotherapy regimen to knock it into remission, several rounds of additional chemotherapy, and a bone marrow transplant. Then there would be everything else—prolonged hospitalizations for expected and unexpected complications, dozens of new pills, learning to live with a weakened immune system, indwelling catheters, blood transfusions, scans, bone marrow biopsies, and many, many doctor's appointments. It is impossible—and probably ill advised—to convey all that in the first meeting. My own philosophy is to dole it out in pieces.

Planning a patient's treatment requires an understanding of his whole situation. Jin's white blood cell count was relevant, of course, but so were factors like where he lived, who lived with him, what his level of independence was, what a typical day was like for him, and what mattered to him.

Planning also requires understanding that plans change. Jin's medical story would evolve over time. He was charting a course whose outline I could see, but with twists and turns expected.

Jin had the good sense to ask one of the most vital questions right away: who is my doctor? His lack of insurance muddied the question, and I knew it would take a village to help answer it. As the oncology fellow on the leukemia ward, every day at 1:20 p.m. I ran a multidisciplinary team meeting. The charge nurse, case manager, social worker, pharmacist, dietitian, physical therapist, scheduler, and I stood in a small circle and ran through our list of shared patients. The purpose of this meeting was to plan—beginning the day a patient is admitted to the hospital—what happens after he leaves.

I started by telling the group that Jin had no health insurance. They all reacted.

"We could send him back to China," the case manager suggested. She did some googling on her phone, pointing out a medical center near his home address. I looked over her shoulder as she pulled up an online flight aggregator. "It would only be one stop," she noted. As we spoke the words aloud, an offhand comment somehow morphing into an itinerary, I realized this plan was absurd. He could bleed. He could become septic. I shook my head. It would be weeks before Jin had a safe window for travel.

Meanwhile, Jin himself took the news in stride. Back in the emergency room, I focused on the part I knew well: the medical next steps. Yes, this was leukemia, and it looked like a type called acute myeloid leukemia. It's a cancer that starts in the bone marrow, the body's factory that produces red blood cells, white blood cells, and platelets. I explained how the disease progresses rapidly and was as serious as it gets, but a cure was possible.

Chasing that cure would mean getting admitted to the hospital and starting chemotherapy right away. The chemotherapy would kill cancerous cells but also kill normal blood cells, so he would be dependent on blood transfusions. Having low blood cell counts weakens the immune system, and many patients develop fevers and are treated for infection. Up to 5 percent of patients die during induction chemotherapy.

Jin and Vanessa asked me the same questions most people do. How long have I had this? (I can't say for sure but likely just a few weeks.) How did my father get this? (This was nothing he did or didn't do. It was bad luck—a genetic mistake.) Will I lose my hair? (Yes, but it will grow back.)

Vanessa and Jin squeezed hands. Then Jin spoke. "I understand," the interpreter translated. "I want the treatment."

I nodded. Next I got into the nitty-gritty. We would perform a bone marrow biopsy. We would do an echocardiogram of his heart and place an indwelling catheter into his arm. We would start him on a pill, taken twice per day, to lower his white blood count. We would give him fluids through his IV and another pill to prevent tumor lysis syndrome, a phenomenon where cancerous cells burst open and can damage organs like the kidneys.

He would stay in the hospital for a total of three to four weeks. "Why so long?" Vanessa wanted to know. "Because we expect complications," I said. "We need to be close enough to react to them."

In Jin's case, they started right away.

LIKE IT OR NOT, taking into account all angles of a patient's story includes the financial ones. My patients' health insurance plans are plastered on the front of their electronic charts. It's one of the first things I look at, right up there with their name and age. I've learned to initiate prior authorizations—a strange process where I have to convince an insurance company that a test I ordered or a treatment I prescribed is necessary. I then get on the phone and do an even more bizarre thing called a peer-to-peer, where I make my case to someone who is not my patient's doctor and sometimes not even a practicing doctor at all. I've learned to finesse phrasing in my notes to guarantee both medical accuracy and maximize the odds of insurance approval. When all else fails, I've also learned to redirect patients to more affordable options.

At its most basic level, having health insurance in this country is synonymous to access—to doctors, hospitals, and medical services such as tests, procedures, and prescriptions. Most Americans obtain health insurance through their work, a practice that was set up during World War II. The country faced a labor shortage as workers were diverted to military duty, and the government worried that raising wages to attract workers would worsen inflation as the nation emerged from the Depression. So in 1942 the Stabilization Act was passed to limit businesses' ability to raise wages. In practice it led employers to adopt alternate incentives to woo workers, such as health insurance. In 1943 the Internal Revenue Service decided employer contributions to health insurance premiums were tax free, further incentivizing the practice. Employer-sponsored health insurance remains the norm to this day. Those who don't have it rely on government-sponsored programs such as Medicare and Medicaid and individual insurance options.

Still, a substantial minority of Americans remain uninsured and underinsured, meaning their plans are insufficient to cover the cost of the medical care they need. One of the main goals of the Affordable Care Act, passed in 2010, was to reduce this number through incentives, mandates, or both. And it did, with the uninsured population dropping from more than 48 million in 2010 to 30 million in 2020. But that still leaves close to 10 percent of the nation without coverage, and costs remain prohibitive even for many who have it.

An ongoing debate in our political discourse is the extent of the moral element to this story: that is, do people have a right to receive medical care regardless of their ability to pay? We as a nation decided that in certain circumstances the answer is a definitive yes: in 1986 a federal act called the Emergency Medical Treatment and Labor Act (EMTALA) was passed. It required anyone coming to an emergency department to be stabilized and treated regardless of insurance status. (Still, an obligation to treat doesn't mean an obligation to treat for free—meaning after emergency care, patients can receive an exorbitant bill.)

What comes next is the part where the law gets blurrier. After a patient is treated for an emergency, does EMTALA require provision of follow-up care regardless of insurance status? Here the answer is sometimes yes. A patient who gets stitches can be seen for suture removal. A patient whose broken bone has been set in a cast can get follow-up X-rays and removal of the cast. In some cases, follow-up care applies to hospitalizations, too. If you're sick enough to be hospitalized, the logic goes, that's sick enough to be considered an emergency. This means we were obligated, not just by our sense of morality but by the law, to treat Jin's complications in the hospital until he was safe enough to leave.

But then what? There is no EMTALA for additional follow-up. What that means, practically, is that hospitals can't turn away a patient whose life is threatened by a newly diagnosed leukemia, but they can turn him away for the chemotherapy that would provide a long-term cure. We can't turn away a patient with a serious diabetic ulceration, but we can turn him away to manage the medications that would have prevented it. The law requires that we douse the fire, but so long as a patient is uninsured or underinsured, we are limited in taking the steps to prevent it from bursting into flames in the first place.

BUT OF COURSE things burst into flames; chronic illness is the kindling. Jin Wong's kindling was leukemia. Any oncologist knows the disease is flammable enough to keep a patient in the hospital for nearly a month during the first round of intensive chemotherapy, as I recommended to Jin and Vanessa. Any oncologist also knows that it's nonsensical to pretend the emergency is over after a month.

When I presented Jin's case to our full medical team the next morning, one of the resident's ears perked up. The resident—I'll call him Vivek—was interested in oncology, and he wanted to learn how to perform bone marrow biopsies on his own. I would train Vivek the same way I had learned: see one, do one, teach one.

After he observed me perform one bone marrow biopsy, we went to Jin's room. We helped Jin turn onto his stomach. I reviewed with Vivek how to palpate the hip bone to mark the right spot. We slipped on our gowns and sterile gloves. We cleaned the skin with an antiseptic solution and covered it with a sterile drape. We drew up 5 milliliters of lidocaine, a local anesthetic, and injected it through the skin, through the subcutaneous tissue, and to the edge of the bone. We used a scalpel to nick a small incision. I handed Vivek a bone marrow aspiration needle, and he pushed through the incision. Then he stopped. "Do you feel bone?" I asked. "I think so," he said. He clenched his hand around the grip and applied pressure. He twisted the needle—back and forth, back and forth, as he chiseled inward. Once the needle was tethered, we connected it to an empty syringe. Vivek pulled back. I expected to see the syringe fill with dark red liquid, but there was nothing. He let go and pulled back again—still nothing.

Vivek looked at me—now what? "We try again," I said. We pulled out the needle, repalpated the hip bone, and identified a spot slightly to the left of his first attempt. We talked through the steps aloud once more. Then he gripped the needle and took another stab. He twisted and pushed. He drew back on the syringe again as a few pink bubbles sputtered up. I shook my head: it wasn't enough.

The incision on Jin's hip was now oozing, and a small pool of blood gathered over the drape. "Let's hold pressure, then try for the biopsy," I said, pressing gauze and referring to the next part of the procedure that takes a solid chunk of marrow. When the bleeding slowed, Vivek went back in. He twisted and pushed. By this point, beads of sweat had pooled on his forehead, and we still had no sample. But I remembered the oncology fellow who taught me: had she taken over when I struggled, I never would have learned.

Jin said something then. Vivek stopped, the biopsy needle halfway wedged. I looked at Vanessa, who was sitting in the corner of the room. She translated, "My chest hurts."

"Where does it hurt?" I asked.

"The left," Jin answered.

I didn't like that. But he didn't have any shortness of breath, the pain didn't radiate to his shoulder or jaw, and he was lying on his chest, after all. We helped him shift to a different position, and I asked Jin if he could stay that way for just a few more minutes. "Yes," he said.

We had to go fast, which meant doing the biopsy myself. I slipped on a fresh pair of sterile gloves. I felt the landmarks, numbed a new patch of skin, and sliced a new incision. I pushed the biopsy needle through and felt bone. I anchored down and twisted. As I began to sweat myself, I thought that Vivek started with a tough one. I felt a gentle pop as I anchored the needle and connected it to a clean syringe. I pulled back: the dark red marrow was slow but flowing. It would be enough.

We peeled off our gowns and gloves and helped Jin turn on his back. But even after the pressure on his chest was relieved, he couldn't get comfortable. "My chest hurts," he said again.

To be safe, I placed orders for an ECG and a blood test called a troponin that would screen for problems with his heart. Then we went upstairs to the last patient. This time Vivek slid the needle into the bone easily. He pulled out a centimeter-long solid piece of marrow that he dropped triumphantly into a petri dish.

When we were done, I checked the computer for the ECG and troponin results on Jin. Both were normal. I checked his vital signs: also normal. I went back to his room and asked the bedside nurse if he was still complaining of chest pain. "He mentioned it once," she said. I looked through the doorway and saw Jin was napping.

After a certain amount of time as a doctor, you develop a kind of sixth sense for trouble, even in the face of objective evidence. It doesn't tell you exactly what's wrong but guides the answer to the question: is this something or nothing? It's the feeling that makes you go back to see a patient napping comfortably, even when there's empirically nothing wrong but your gut saying there is. It was the feeling that made me order another ECG and troponin on Jin to be done in six hours.

Around midnight I was awakened at home by the high-pitched beep of my pager. When I called back, both the on-call cardiology fellow and overnight medicine resident were on the line. Jin's troponin had jumped up. His ECG showed abnormal depressions. His oxygen had fallen, and he was now requiring six supplemental liters through a full face mask.

We talked through the possibilities that could explain this sudden constellation of findings. Was it a myocardial infarction (heart attack) or a pulmonary embolism (blood clot in the lungs)? Could it be leukostasis (a phenomenon where white blood cells glom together and clog critical vessels)?

Jin was sick enough that we had to treat the most dangerous possibilities. Another thought entered my mind that I wished I could push out: this is going to cost a lot. When I spoke to Jin and Vanessa about costs earlier, Jin had guided me: "Do whatever you think is best, doctor." I recalled those words and realized how vague they actually were—best for him how? Medically, personally, financially? If only those goals aligned.

I had to decide. "Let's transfer him to the ICU," I told the overnight resident. Then I slipped on my scrubs and got in my car.

IN THE NEXT TWENTY-FOUR HOURS, Jin's team of doctors tripled, the cost of his hospitalization skyrocketed, and his medical complexities and prescriptions multiplied.

Jin woke up in a chilly, white-walled room. A central line that he'd consented to amid a blur of scrubs and white coats had been inserted into his neck. He now tried to tug on it. A nurse grabbed his hand. No, she shook her head, and Jin didn't need an interpreter to understand that he should stop.

Overnight we performed apheresis through Jin's catheter to filter out the excess white blood cells. The ICU team called me the next morning to go on rounds with them. There was now an ICU attending, a daytime resident and a daytime fellow (both different from the overnight ones), and a different cardiology fellow. Jin scanned the sea of unfamiliar faces and noticeably relaxed when he saw me. "My doctor!" he pointed. Everyone smiled. It really was sweet.

An echocardiogram that afternoon showed part of Jin's heart ballooning out, weakening its ability to pump. Even though his vital signs and labs were improving, Jin's weakened heart meant we could no longer give the chemotherapy we had planned. So we spoke to Jin and Vanessa about switching to a regimen that was safer for the heart, consisting of one intravenous infusion and one pill.

The good news was that the heart failure would likely completely resolve with time. The bad news was that Jin's multiplying complexities meant that follow-up would be more important than ever. So I continued to run our daily 1:20 p.m. meetings to plan for it. I learned from my team that Jin couldn't be seen in our oncology clinic without agreeing to pay for the visit out of pocket; with his follow-up no longer deemed an emergency, EMTALA didn't apply. In turn, I shared the latest complication with the group as they scrambled to update their planning. The pharmacist asked how many pills of the new chemotherapy he would need. The case manager wanted to know how long the indwelling catheter would remain.

To devise an affordable plan, every team member asked the same question: what will Jin *need*? My job was to predict those needs, à la carte: venetoclax (a drug used to fight the leukemia), let's say for a year; furosemide (a diuretic that would relieve fluid accumulation from heart failure), I'll guess for two months; oh, and blood work would have to be checked twice weekly because he will continue to need blood transfusions. And an echocardiogram, let's plan for a month from now. The furosemide could alter his electrolytes, so he will need potassium supplements, or it could mess with his fluid status, and in that case he'd need . . .

Predicting the details of Jin's medical course to try to lock down what he would need was an exercise in futility. What he needed was a regular doctor who could respond to these developments in real time. Jin's team worked valiantly behind the scenes to secure him a year's worth of chemotherapy pills free of charge from the company who made them. They convinced the hospital to absorb a large chunk of the cost of his hospital care. It was incredible to be a part of this group, and yet there was only so much we could do. Assembling a group of health care professionals to navigate the fragmentation imposed by health insurance felt as roundabout as hiring extra staff to manage the electronic charts.

In the absence of secured follow-up, what can an uninsured or underinsured patient do? Some turn to the emergency room (even after the Affordable Care Act was passed, in 2016 nearly one in ten emergency room visits involved uninsured patients), a messy nonsolution that emergency rooms are unequipped to handle. Some patients decide to pay out of pocket and try to negotiate in advance what services they need most—a recipe discordant with medicine's twists and turns. Alternatively, they can turn to what we call the health care safety net—a patchwork of programs and providers including county hospital systems and free clinics that serve people with low incomes, no insurance coverage, or other special needs.

Starting in 2016, I spent some Saturdays volunteering to supervise medical students in a local free clinic. The clinic was located about thirty miles from the hospital where I usually worked, and as I pulled into the parking lot for the first time, I realized that it was actually a high school. Handwritten signs next to the tennis courts pointed me to classrooms doubling as medical exam rooms. As medical students presented cases to me, I struggled to figure out what exactly we could do for these patients. I learned that with limited resources and rotating physician volunteers, this was not a place for regular follow-up. The goal, much like in the emergency room, was to do any transaction that was possible (suture a wound, prescribe antibiotics, order some tests). The bigger goal was then to connect the patient to a regular doctor elsewhere in the safety net.

One Saturday morning I met a soft-spoken elderly couple from Nigeria who crystallized for me just how limited my role was. They came with a few specific complaints: her vision was blurry, and he couldn't stop urinating. I asked some questions and examined them both, and by the end of the visit I believed that she had cataracts and was concerned that he might have prostate cancer. Had they been insured, the next step for the wife would have been a referral to an eye doctor. For her husband, I would have ordered urine testing and a blood test called a PSA (prostate-specific antigen), with the next step being a possible prostate biopsy. But here I wasn't sure what to do. We can do the urine tests and PSA, I offered, recommending that he come back to go over the results with another doctor. But what if they were suggestive of prostate cancer? The layers of follow-up needed were daunting—and unavailable.

The health care safety net is better than nothing. Those who work there are among the kindest and most dedicated souls you can find. But the safety net is still just that: a net. A net catches. A net reacts. A net has holes.

The patients I saw in the free clinic were often medically complex because they had delayed seeing a doctor for years. Diabetes ran unchecked. Tumors grew to the size of grapefruits. What I saw was the end result of a system that didn't care for people until it reached the point of emergency. What these patients needed was beyond what any high school doubling as a health care center could offer in one or two visits. What we could offer was transactional, reactive, and piecemeal: a quick fix to a contained problem. Most patients disappeared into the chasm that I got used to charting as "lost to follow-up."

I learned that one of the most valuable things I could do here was convey this to patients. Just as I developed a speech imploring my patients to obtain their own medical records and advocate for their stories, I developed another about how vital it is to find a primary doctor. I told the couple from Nigeria just how little we could accomplish in a one-time visit. I explained that regular, consistent access to a doctor you can afford is better than fragmented, sporadic access to one you cannot. I offered them resources on how to get insured. I relayed how to look for a primary doctor in the county clinic. Tears filled their eyes, and my heart broke as I saw how grateful they were for what felt like so little.

I thought about them as I discussed Jin with the leukemia attending, a doctor I'll call Dave. Dave suddenly had an idea. He remembered the name of a doctor he knew from fellowship who now worked at a county hospital about an hour south. Dave pulled out his phone and was happy to find he still had this person's cell phone number. I wrote it down, and then I cold-called him.

"I can tell you more details," I started. "But right now what we need most is someone to follow up."

I could tell that the doctor on the line was a caring person. He listened and was sympathetic, but he didn't have the capacity to accept new patients right now, he told me. He passed on the names of two colleagues at the county hospital who also saw uninsured patients with cancer. Maybe one of them could become Jin's doctor?

I thanked him. I called both other office numbers and spoke to receptionists. One doctor had left the county hospital, and the other "didn't treat leukemia anymore." I hung up the phone, deflated.

Someone had to follow up. But who?

JUST AS OUR FEDERAL LAW doesn't appreciate the importance of medical follow-up, I didn't always appreciate it either. During my first few years as a doctor, I was drawn to high-acuity, high-stakes situations. I thrived on being able to manipulate machines and drips to keep a person alive. I loved having the expertise to run up to a crashing patient, command a room, and turn the tide on a dire situation. I loved the evolution from feeling my heart race and then slow in medical emergencies, being in control and clear-eyed in crisis. This felt like real medicine to me.

Those moments are powerful, but they're more powerful when they're not just moments. In the clinic some of my most rewarding saves involved incremental, positive change over time: helping a patient quit smoking, diagnosing coronary artery disease and getting someone on the right medications *before* the crushing chest pain, and managing side effects from chemotherapy regimens and weighing the tradeoffs of continuing them. I started to feel an even bigger thrill in playing the long game; it felt like playing chess to keep my patients well.

But similar to retrieving records or adding up potassium levels, long-term relationships with patients were not something the system easily allowed. As I rotated through hospital wards and clinics, establishing short bursts of meaningful relationships and then saying goodbye, I created workarounds to make the continuity happen.

Shortly before meeting Jin, I was the oncology fellow called about a fifty-something-year-old woman who had experienced two weeks of low-grade fevers and night sweats. The inpatient medicine team ordered a PET scan, which lit up with enlarged lymph nodes in her neck, chest, and abdomen. To help figure out why, they called a cadre of specialists: the infectious diseases doctor, the rheumatologist, and me.

I recommended a biopsy of one of the lymph nodes in her neck to evaluate for lymphoma or another cancer. The team did one, and it was inconclusive. So we tried to biopsy another enlarged node and got the same result.

The only remaining option was to biopsy a lymph node in her abdomen, but this wasn't easy to reach with a needle. The medicine team spoke to the on-call general surgeon, who said it would take a laparotomy to get to it.

This is no small matter. A laparotomy is a full-blown operation under general anesthesia. It requires a multi-inch abdominal incision, carries risks of surgical complications, and takes weeks to heal. "But if you need it, we'll do it," the surgeon said. I was hesitant to give the green light. This wasn't necessarily a lymphoma; it was not uncommon to see enlarged lymph nodes from some kind of viral infection, even if the infectious diseases team couldn't pinpoint one. I was reassured that the patient's fevers and night sweats were already abating. At the same time, I wouldn't want a possible cancer to grow unchecked. I trudged through her test results, looking for clues that would push me one way or another.

Finally, I proposed a compromise: order and review another

PET scan in one month. There was only one piece missing. Who would follow up on the scan?

The patient had no regular doctor. I walked over to the lymphoma clinic and asked if anyone there could see her in follow-up. No, not without a diagnosis, I was told; we can't go around filling up our schedule with people who don't have biopsy-proven cancer. I referred her to a primary care clinic within her insurance network, but I knew it might fall through: the drive was far, and the co-pays, even within network, were prohibitively high.

I was off the hospital consult service by the time the PET scan was done, but I felt I had no choice. I added her to a follow-up list I created for myself. One month later I pulled up the scan from my home computer. The enlarged nodes were resolved, validating our decision to watch and wait.

I called the number we had on file. "Hi, Ms. L?"

"Yes?"

"This is Dr. Yurkiewicz. I don't know if you remember me, but . . ."

"I remember you. What did my scan show? Do I need the biopsy?"

I treated another patient in the hospital for diffuse muscle and joint aches whom we diagnosed with an autoimmune condition. Her recovery would take time, so we discharged her to a rehab facility with intensive physical, occupational, and speech therapy. We started new medications, including pain medications for her body aches.

Again there was only one problem. Someone needed to keep close tabs on the meds and on her. She had a doctor listed in her chart as her primary, but "I only met her once, and I didn't like her very much," she told me. I felt the familiar void, like driving across a bridge and seeing it dissolve before my eyes. She pressed me, and reluctantly I gave her my cell phone number. The next day she called me in a frenzy. She was hours overdue for pain medication, and she hadn't seen a doctor yet. I called over and left a message for the rehab doctor. But the truth was the moment she stepped out the hospital front doors, I was no longer her doctor, and I had no real power over her care. All I could do was make suggestions.

The closest I got to successful continuity of care was with a retired scientist who suffered from severe scoliosis and decided to go ahead with an elective operation called a spinal fusion to straighten it. But in the operating room, she lost liters of blood and had a cardiac arrest on the table. She survived but only after weeks in the ICU on dialysis and a ventilator.

I was the internal medicine doctor in the hospital who accepted her as she was transferred from the ICU to the wards. Her legs were puffy and her abdomen distended. Her heart kept flipping in and out of an arrhythmia. A litany of medications was carried over from the ICU, including cardiac medications, diuretics, antianxiety meds, pain pills, sleep meds, constipation meds, and blood thinners. I wrote a list cataloging my assessment and plan for addressing each medical problem. All of this would need to be sorted out and dealt with over time to optimize her recovery.

As I made careful progress on fixing her medical conditions over the next two weeks, she and I grew close in the hospital. When she was well enough to leave, she was understandably nervous. I thought I had the perfect solution; as a resident at the time, I was in a unique position because I saw patients in both the hospital and the clinic. So I handed her my business card and asked her to see me in my clinic, which was in her insurance network. This would be a handoff from myself to myself.

For a few months, the benefits were clear. By knowing her medical story inside and out, I could continue charting a long-term path toward recovery. One time she came to my clinic so sleepy that she dozed off as we were speaking. Had I not known her, it would have been easy to think she looked too sick to be home and to admit her to the hospital. But I knew better because I knew her.

I asked a few questions and changed a few things. Her abdominal distension indicated she was severely constipated, and I prescribed a stronger enema. I also halved her sleep medications. By the next day she was fine.

But after a few months, the situation became harder. "It takes us over an hour to get here in traffic," her husband said. I could hear the exhaustion in both their voices. Close follow-up meant, well, following up closely; for a while I was seeing her every few weeks. "I'm just being realistic," her husband said one day. "We need someone closer to home."

I gave them a few names and hoped she found a new doctor, but when I looked at her chart a year later, I saw she hadn't. There had been no shortage of appointments, but they were all with specialists, many for one-time visits. Who was directing her overall story, working on chronic pain, constipation, sleep, fluid overload, hypertension, and heart failure? I had no answer. The chart also showed me she was back to being hospitalized frequently. I wondered how many of those hospital stays could have been avoided with careful, familiar follow-up.

I KNEW THAT IF JIN FOLLOWED THE SAME PATH, the results could be catastrophic, but we still had no solution. After he was well enough to leave the hospital, he agreed to pay over a thousand dollars out of pocket to see me and Dave in the clinic. Two weeks later, we sat together in the exam room as we checked his blood counts, transfused one unit of platelets, stopped one of his heart medications, and prescribed a preventive antifungal medication and antibiotic. We advised him and Vanessa to buy a home thermometer and reinforced that anything greater than 100.4 degrees Fahrenheit should prompt a trip back to the emergency room.

One week later, Jin began to cough at home. Vanessa took his temperature, remembered our words, and drove him to the emergency room. He was evaluated by the emergency doctors and admitted to the leukemia team, which by this point had rotated to a different attending, different fellow, and different residents. They started him on IV antibiotics and ordered a CT scan of his chest, which showed patchy infiltrates in both lungs. The infectious disease team was summoned, and a crowd of new doctors formed. Jin asked the infectious disease doctors about the state of his leukemia, and they deferred to his leukemia team. He asked his leukemia team, who deferred bigger-picture questions to his primary oncologist.

I had rotated off the leukemia wards and was off from work altogether that day. But when I heard from the new fellow that Jin was back, I drove to the hospital. The nurses I knew well didn't recognize me at first when I headed toward his room in sweatpants and a wrinkly college T-shirt: "Excuse me, who are you visiting? Oh! Hi, Dr. Yurkiewicz!" I sat with Jin and Vanessa, and we talked. I related all the details: "As your team probably told you, you have bacteria in your blood that most likely came from pneumonia. You are receiving IV antibiotics, and they will switch you to oral antibiotics before you leave the hospital. We will decide in the clinic when to stop these. But the good news," I emphasized, "is the leukemia. Your bone marrow showed that it is in remission."

With his intake to the county clinic still in flux, Jin came into our clinic one more time, agreed to pay out of pocket once again, and saw the doctors he knew well.

In the exam room, he smiled broadly. So did I because he was looking better. His energy was up, and his cough had improved. He was able to walk a few blocks around the neighborhood, he said, without feeling winded. But his neutrophils, a type of white blood cell that protects against bacterial infections, were still low, so we planned to delay the next round of chemotherapy for a week.

Our conversation eventually circled around to follow-up. With a period of medical stability, Jin could theoretically go home to China, but Vanessa hesitated. "I can't imagine him going back," she said. Her father lived all alone there. She asked a lot of good questions. Was the county hospital chemo set up? Or would they pay for another cycle here? Who would they call if something went wrong?

WHO IS YOUR DOCTOR? In 2019 three doctors and researchers published a study in a major medical journal where they defined having a primary doctor as being able to answer yes to four questions:

- *Do you have a usual source of care for new health problems?*
- *Do you have a usual source for preventive health care?*
- *Do you have a usual source for referrals?*
- *Do you have a usual source for ongoing health problems?*

One in four Americans do not have this person, the study authors reported one year later. And this number is going in the wrong direction.

Primary care physicians are not the only doctors who provide crucial, ongoing follow-up. Patients with chronic illnesses rely on specialists who are just as instrumental in seeing their patients over time: oncologists manage patients with cancer over years. Rheumatologists care for patients with autoimmune conditions that flare up and go quiescent. Neurologists manage illnesses that can chronically affect quality of life. For all these physicians where follow-up is critical, the data sadly tell the same story: patients struggle to access them, and cost is a big reason why.

Even for patients who are well insured, follow-up is given short shrift. When I began in practice as an attending, I spent hours in orientation learning about how to bill insurance companies for my encounters with patients. I learned that if I saw a new patient, the reimbursement from insurance companies could be twice as high as if I saw a patient in follow-up. For doctors this is a financial acknowledgment that evaluating a new patient involves more cognitive horsepower than assessing someone we know well. But what we have created—for the insured, uninsured, and under-insured—is a health care system where follow-up is downgraded compared to transactional, one-and-done medicine. As long as access is doled out à la carte, there is going to be a ranking of what kind of medical care matters most. This ranking favors acuity over the long term, reacting to sickness over promoting wellness, and interchangeable doctors over relationships.

But this system operates on a fundamental misunderstanding of how medicine works. It works when all of it is thought through, monitored, titrated, coordinated, and changed over time and based on the situation at hand. A trip to the emergency room doesn't do that. A hospitalization doesn't do that. Even "a" doctor cannot do that well. The same doctor does.

Jin Wong never got that doctor. Two weeks later, he was sitting in his recliner at home when he felt unwell. He was weak. He could hardly stand up. He called Vanessa, who was out running errands. "My chest hurts," he told her, a terrifying echo of his earliest complication. She rushed back. First she tried calling the general hospital number, but when the operator asked who she wanted to page, she wasn't sure. She was put on hold and then became entangled in a phone tag until frustration won out and she hung up.

They bundled Jin into the car. It was rush hour, and Vanessa worried that they'd get stuck in traffic on the way to our hospital. So she drove to the closest emergency room, located in a small community hospital a few miles away. The emergency doctor drew blood, ordered an ECG, and shot a chest X-ray. He couldn't identify a primary doctor to call for more background, so he paged the on-call hematology fellow at our hospital. This was a doctor who had never met Jin, but she skimmed his electronic chart and passed off as much information as she could. The emergency doctor then called a local hematologist, a cardiologist, and a pulmonologist. They all agreed to admit Jin to the hospital, start broad antibiotics, and run additional tests on his heart.

I worry the nuances of his medical story were dropped. I worry that despite these doctors' expertise, efforts, and best intentions, meeting Jin anew that night meant something was lost. I don't like to imagine how Jin reacted to it all—seeing all new faces, feeling uncertain, and not knowing where to direct his questions.

Suddenly Jin went limp, and a nurse noticed he wasn't breathing. He had no pulse. A code blue was called. A cavalry of providers ran into the room to try to resuscitate him. After thirty minutes of chest compressions and electric shocks, his pulse never returned. The notes declared his time of death. Vanessa declined an autopsy.

I spoke to her by phone a few days later. I was quiet for a long time as she told me what happened. She didn't blame anyone; instead she thanked me. She told me my relationship with her dad mattered. I told her it mattered to me, too. Mostly she grieved, openly over the phone, as I held it to my ear and cried silently.

I don't know exactly what caused Jin's death. Despite many obstacles, many doctors cared for him as best as they could. But I do know how much gets lost when follow-up is fragmented. I do know how much better I can be as a doctor when I can see my patients regularly. Jin's story pains me deeply. He had an abundance of doctors and yet somehow slid between them. He was in limbo, always looking at faces there to help him, each reacting expertly when something went wrong. All the while, he lacked the primary doctor to forge the path ahead.

Reform will come when we recognize that seeing a regular doctor isn't optional and it isn't a luxury. Fixing what went wrong in Jin's story will take prioritizing the slow, meticulous, ordinary, crucial, life-saving work of follow-up.

JIN ASKED ME MANY HARD QUESTIONS during the two months we shared. He wanted to know how long he had to live. He wanted to know what it would feel like to die. We would speak for long periods as I walked the tightrope between being as candid as I could while acknowledging the uncertainty inherent in predicting. But there's one question to which I keep returning.

It was our first meeting in the emergency room, and our conversation was winding down. "Do you have any other questions?" I had asked.

Jin reached over and took both my hands in his. "You are my doctor from now on," the interpreter translated. "Right?"

"Well, yes and no," I stammered. I fumbled the answer to what should have been the simplest question. It wasn't simple at all.

Chapter 5

Twenty-Eight Hours in Hell

WHEN I WAS PAGED ABOUT JIN WONG AT MIDNIGHT, I drove back to the hospital without hesitation, even though I had been working all day and I would be working all the next day as well. Jin was my patient, and I was compelled by a doctor's sense of responsibility for her patients. But I also went in because of a schedule laid out for me: I was the doctor on call.

The part of the story I glossed over earlier was how I felt the next day. By late morning, I finished rounds on all my patients including Jin. By early afternoon, I slunk to a call room to squeeze in a quick power nap. Just as I was drifting off, my pager blared, I had missed multiple secure text messages, and my phone was ringing. There were patients to be seen, work to be done.

It is no secret that doctors work extreme hours. Occasionally I have introduced myself as someone's new doctor, only to have him eye me up and down and ask, "What hour are you on?" During my residency and fellowship, which encompassed my first six years as a doctor, a typical work week consisted of eighty hours in the hospital. My standard number of workdays per week was six (doctors call a full weekend off a "golden weekend," while for most people I realize this is simply called a "weekend"). And in my world, being on call is all encompassing. It is nothing like the TV portrayal showing someone out or relaxing at home before the pager beeps to signal the character is a doctor. Being on call in real life is jam-packed and relentless; often you never have the chance to go home.

Perhaps the most controversial feature of a doctor's schedule is the shift of twenty-eight consecutive hours—a staple of residency and fellowship programs in most hospitals across the country. Residents in the broadest specialties, such as internal medicine and general surgery, spend at least a few months working these hours every three to four days. Just how long twenty-eight hours actually is became clear during one of my residency shifts in the ICU when a friend was in town for a day. She asked in a text, would I be free for lunch or dinner? Can't, I replied. She was in town for one more day: how about breakfast the next day or coffee after that? She named subsequent meals that in a normal world represented different slices of time. But 8:00 a.m. one day to noon the next was all the same for me—hours bleeding together, my sense of time warped, and the entirety of my surroundings contained in the fluorescent box of the ICU. During another especially busy call, I remember looking at my watch after twelve exhausting hours had passed. I realized with horror that *I still had sixteen to go.* I became an ant during these shifts: don't look too far ahead; take it one breadcrumb at a time.

To work these hours effectively, you develop tricks that arise from intimately getting to know your body's limitations. I had my night-before, wind-down rituals to make sure I could lull myself into a full eight hours of sleep before heading into a twenty-eight-hour stretch. I learned to stagger my caffeinated beverages at just the right times to keep me alert but not jittery. I learned how to nap in strange places and even stranger positions (once I fell asleep standing up). During these shifts, I tucked syringes of urgent medications in my front scrub pocket and kept laminated checklists in my back pocket. My goal was to keep my body and surroundings as optimized as possible to compensate for what I knew was coming: mental lapses that escalated with each passing hour.

When I reached the end of my twenty-eight hours, my head hurt, my feet ached, and I never got behind a steering wheel. But in the face of the immense suffering our patients experience, it can feel tactless to complain about ourselves. I knew that my discomfort, which was curable with a nap, was a mosquito bite in the face of true suffering. I felt privileged to be immersed in work that mattered and humbled to help others at their most vulnerable. I also know what it's like to be on the other side of the stethoscope, not sleeping for nights on end as a loved one teeters between life and death. There is no contest as to which is worse.

But refusing to acknowledge the harmful effects of these hours because it could be worse is a trap. Having worked these shifts many times, as well as standard hours, I have seen clearly that there is nothing intrinsic to being a doctor that requires such harshness. Doing good work as a doctor and working reasonable hours is a false dichotomy.

And yet shifts lasting twenty-four or more consecutive hours have been a fixture in medicine for decades. They persist because of one unrelenting argument, which postures itself as one of combating fragmentation: longer hours, it is said, are better for fostering ongoing relationships between doctors and patients. In 2017 the Accreditation Council for Graduate Medical Education (ACGME), the organization responsible for setting restrictions on work hours in residency, removed all prohibitions against working twenty-eight consecutive hours as a way of "re-establishing the commitment to team-based care and seamless continuity of care." Framed this way, the logic borders on the obvious: continuous hours lead to continuous medical care. A doctor working many hours in a row can manage their patients' medical stories without the gaps that would result from leaving and coming back, the reasoning goes.

Many have pushed back, lamenting the effects of sleep deprivation on doctors' health. Others have condemned these hours by pointing out how fatigue worsens cognition, harming doctors' ability to make sound decisions. (Being awake more than twenty-four hours is like having a blood alcohol content of 0.1 percent, above the threshold for being considered legally drunk, the studies tell us.) I am sympathetic to both lines of reasoning, and arguments can certainly be made to abolish these shifts for these reasons alone.

Yet there is even more going on here. It's not just the long hours that are harmful; it's how those hours are spent. The continuity that is constantly invoked to justify these shifts is a myth. In fact, the opposite is true.

IT IS 1:00 A.M., and I am losing patience. This is a suboptimal emotion for a doctor responsible for the lives of the sickest patients in the hospital. I am wearing sterile garb and am hunched over the radial artery of a woman in shock. I position my ultrasound over the cold gel on her wrist with one hand and steady my needle with the other. I need to place an arterial line to monitor her bottoming-out blood pressure, which is only stable because of the vasopressor drips I have running through her veins. But I can't get the needle in. The artery spasms, its silhouette on the ultrasound screen collapsing. It's too small for my needle.

As I think about how to troubleshoot this problem, a nurse pokes her head in. "The room next door, with the new patient," she starts. "I promise I'll be there soon," I say. "I'm almost done here."

The year was 2017, and I was a senior resident working twenty-eight-hour shifts every four days in the ICU. The intervening days were regular workdays—from 6:00 a.m. to 5:00 p.m. We worked as a team of four resident doctors, meaning during the day one doctor was home sleeping, one was starting the first half of her twenty-eight hours, and the other two were working routine shifts. During overnight call, I was glued to what we called the

"Batphone," everyone else's cherished lifeline to the on-call ICU doctor. But for the person carrying the phone, the temptation to throw it against a wall was ever-present. All day and all night, it rang. I could be in the midst of resuscitating one patient who was crashing only to have to field numerous calls from nurses reporting blood gases and specialists getting back with recommendations. On a good night, I could squeeze in an hour or two of napping, but the Batphone was like an interminable alarm clock. To this day, whenever I hear a ringtone even vaguely resembling it, I jolt to attention.

At around 9:00 p.m. that evening, I went from room to room to assess each patient in the ICU. I spoke to each bedside nurse and reviewed ongoing problems as I tried to anticipate questions. This was a script every on-call doctor followed. The goal was to protect any potential sleeping time by tucking away as much work as possible in advance.

Despite this routine, going without sleep is often inevitable because in addition to managing all the current ICU patients, the on-call doctor also manages new admissions. By this time of the night, I have admitted two new patients and am juggling the care of all the others. I am starting to feel the familiar toll of heavy eyelids and impatience with complexity, but there's nothing I can do about it. I must go on.

I somehow manage to insert the arterial line into my patient's wrist. I throw away my sterile gloves and unroll the papers from my back scrub pocket, where I had taken notes on a man I'll call Burt Klein, a seventy-year-old retired teacher I learned would be transferring from another hospital by ambulance.

Two weeks ago, he went to the hospital because of a bad flu and a superimposed bacterial pneumonia. Burt then developed an autoimmune storm—a condition in which a patient's immune system attacks his own organs—that nearly took his life. Diffuse alveolar hemorrhage caused bleeding into his lungs, and after being urgently intubated, the doctors at the other hospital treated him with high-dose steroids and a monoclonal antibody infusion to try to calm his immune system. But his respiratory failure worsened, and he was unable to come off the ventilator. He now has a tracheostomy—a tube inserted in the neck for breathing support—and a feeding tube. He has kidney failure requiring dialysis. Ultrasounds showed blood clots clogging the veins of both legs, but he is not on blood thinners because his platelet counts are critically low. Like most ICU patients, he remains very much in limbo between life and death. And as his doctor, I am tasked with making decisions that have enormous power to sway the outcome one way or the other.

Questions are immediately running through my mind. I start jotting down notes about the possible causes of his kidney failure. (Was his urine spun in a centrifuge and examined under a microscope at the other hospital? Could his kidneys be suffering from the same autoimmune process that harmed his lungs? There was no kidney biopsy done, was there?) I see his platelets are low, and I repeat the process of trying to understand why. (Is the low count due to medications, bone marrow failure, or a destructive autoimmune process? Had the doctors at the other hospital ruled out heparin-induced thrombocytopenia?)

Normally these are patients to whom I am drawn. I prefer complexity—where multiple organs may be involved, the diagnosis remains uncertain, and recovery depends on sound judgment and careful thought about the order of events. I would eagerly grab the stack of papers and dig in.

But after working for seventeen hours straight, I feel like my brain is slogging through quicksand. I remember once hearing a physician describe our skill set in internal medicine as, "Our reasoning is our scalpel." My scalpel is dull.

I introduce myself to Burt and ask if I can examine him. He nods his head up and down. He is on a setting of the ventilator called pressure support, air puffing into his lungs through the plastic tubing in his neck. I place my stethoscope over his lungs and hear faint crackles throughout. His legs, mottled and cool, are covered up to his thighs in dark purple spots. His wife, Patricia, who I learn is also an educator, sits by his bedside. She wears horn-rimmed glasses, and I appreciate her deliberate way of speaking. I wonder if her husband was the same before he fell ill. I imagine them at the dinner table, engaging in respectful, thoughtful conversation. It pierces me to picture how much has changed.

But the clock is ticking, and I can't let myself spend too much time on emotions. I explain the plan for the night to both of them and then flip through his outside records in more detail as I place admission orders on a computer. I start with the basics: ventilator settings, tube feeds, line care, blood checks. I carry over the same dosing of steroids he was receiving at the outside hospital. There is a note in the chart about a misplaced feeding tube right before his respiratory failure worsened. I stop. I make a note to myself to investigate this further. I know all too well that once one piece of the critical illness story becomes most pressing, other things can be forgotten. Was the feeding tube ever moved into the correct location?

These thoughts are interrupted by the incessant ringing of the Batphone. I have admitted a twenty-four-year-old with necrotizing pancreatitis from heavy drinking, a middle-aged man with metastatic cholangiocarcinoma with septic shock from fungus growing in his bloodstream and lungs, and an older woman with cirrhosis who presents with seizures and a gastrointestinal bleed.

Each patient brings a lot to sort through. By the time I come up with plans for the new patients, with frequent detours to put out fires on others, it is almost 5:00 a.m. I head to the call room with its bunkbeds, conveniently located within the ICU. I remove the syringes and my curled-up notes from my scrub pockets and drop them on a tray table that doubles as a nightstand. Just a few minutes, I think, as I climb up to the top bed. I stare at the ceiling for a few minutes, my mind swirling with to-dos. Then I close my eyes.

Barely twenty minutes pass before my break is over. "A new transfer is coming," a nurse shouts into the phone. (I remember it as shouting. I'm sure she was speaking at a perfectly normal decibel level.)

If the intent is "seamless continuity of care," as the ACGME calls it—I don't want to leave my patient in the middle of his case—my shifts raise a question: why am I admitting so many new patients? Rather than preserving continuity over a single case, for many doctors these calls simply pack more work into more hours: more patients, more central lines, more piles of papers dropped onto our desks from other hospitals. Brand-new patients arrived at midnight, 2:00 a.m., 4:00 a.m., and beyond, each needing a workup whether I had been on the job for one hour or twenty-three hours. How seamless is the continuity of care when I admit a new patient at 5:00 a.m. and then pass along his care to a different doctor two hours later?

As the hours pass and my workload grows, it is inevitable; I cut corners. First to go are administrative tasks. A crushing workload shines a spotlight on how much of what you do involves clerical fat; it also gives you a newfound empowerment to trim it. I freely reroute my last vestiges of energy into caring for patients, not tidying their charts. My notes are brief. I update no problem lists. I keep a steady distance from the fax machine.

Next to go is politeness. I refuse to morph into the jerk doctor who snaps at good people just doing their jobs. But there are no extra qualifiers, no small talk, and no soothing of egos. One nurse has called me multiple times over the last few hours about the same patient. The nurse has noticed that the patient is confused. I had ordered a brain MRI at 11:00 p.m. and after review determined it was unchanged from his previous one. Among all my ICU patients, I am least worried about this man, whose confusion has a multitude of causes we are actively treating, but the well-rested nurse who is responsible for him alone continues to bombard me. He bursts into the call room at one point as I try to rest. "The patient is *confused*," he tells me. I ask what he is worried about. He cannot say. Is anything different? "No," he admits. I say that if perhaps we let the patient rest and stop waking him every few hours, he will be less confused. Persistence, advocacy, and open communication—traits I would admire in coworkers in any other situation—are now somehow the enemy.

The last block to fall is speaking with families. I push against this one the hardest, but eventually it becomes impossible. Frightened spouses and other loved ones arrive at all hours of the night, and they want an update. They ask the nurse, "May we speak to the doctor?" I am forced to triage these requests like anything else, and it breaks my heart. If it's not urgent, it can wait until morning. It *must* wait until morning.

One by one, tasks fall by the wayside, tossed aside when they fail to reach a priority threshold I set by necessity. The bare minimum is not the exception but the rule. Nothing about this feels good; it is agonizing to feel like the worst version of yourself when it matters most. But as I juggle a full ICU with its five new admissions, I am preoccupied with what is most pressing in the moment: keeping people alive.

I head back to Burt's room, suddenly remembering the feeding tube. I peel back the dressing and examine the skin around it. I push on his abdomen. Does this hurt? He mouths "no." What about here? He shakes his head from side to side. Reassured, I order a new abdominal X-ray with the morning batch. I file the information about the feeding tube into my note and the back of my brain, and I move on.

Over my last few hours on call, I examine patients and respond to nurses. I insert arterial catheters and interpret lab results. I ultrasound beating hearts. I start antibiotics for one patient who spikes a fever. I start an amiodarone drip for an arrhythmia in another. I perform a death exam on a patient we were managing with comfort measures only, placing my stethoscope on his silent heart and shining a penlight into his unmoving pupils. I offer my condolences to his weeping family at his bedside and don't let myself feel too much—not right now anyway. Every request involves mental triage: What is most urgent? What can wait until an hour from now or until tomorrow?

I am not alone. On the next shift, a different doctor does the same calculus, doing less and less as the hours pass. This raises the question: if we are all ants, focused on the highest-acuity breadcrumbs in front of us, who does the work that's not immediately pressing but just as crucial in the long run? With every shift devolving at some point into skating above the bare minimum, who reads through the four hundred pages of outside hospital records? Who calls the patient's son who speaks a different language? Who sits with the dying patient who has no family by his side?

As the sun rises and the rest of the medical team starts to trickle in, I tell the incoming doctors about my patients from overnight. I join morning rounds, where the entire ICU team discusses each patient, and I relay how I managed the most active patients. Then, while the team moves on to the others, I slink away to a computer. I churn out many, many notes, trying to recollect all my actions and thought processes over a stretch of time that is becoming blurrier by the moment. Close to noon, I vaguely remember walking home. Then I sleep. It is a deep, insistent, overpowering sleep. I dream of vasopressor drips and crash carts. A few hours later, I awaken to a dark evening sky. With a newfound clarity that only rest provides, I think of all the things I could have done differently.

THE STORY OF 28-HOUR SHIFTS is incomplete without detailing what happens on hours 29, 40, 75, and 100. Burt's medical saga didn't end when my eyelids finally closed. As I slept, I missed most of the discussions on morning rounds. That afternoon I dreamed through major changes to the medical plans, discussions with the specialist teams, and family meetings to elucidate end-of-life wishes for loved ones.

I return to the hospital the following morning. A lot has happened, and I have to play catchup. I click through orders and notes, trying to piece together what took place and why from the brief scaffolding hastily typed by another equally exhausted doctor at the end of her shift. Did Mr. R's lumbar puncture results confirm the meningitis I had suspected? Did Ms. S's family opt for comfort care? Often I don't find out the details. The doctor who would know only has the stamina for an abbreviated recap and then goes home to collapse into her own deep sleep.

Every morning the three resident doctors on our team who are conscious divvy up all the patients in the ICU. We try to pair patients with the doctors who know them best, but our scheduling makes this all but impossible. The best I can schedule with Burt is every two or three out of four days.

A few days later, I am discussing the updates to his health on rounds. Respiratory, I say, reviewing Burt's most recent ventilator settings. A different team member pulls up his chest X-ray on the computer screen. I point to the white lines at the bases of both lungs and explain that I gave diuretics to remove extra fluid. The team member then pulls up the X-ray from the previous day and shows the two side by side. "Not that different," the attending doctor says.

"Can you pull up the one from two days before?" I ask. I want to probe the group about something that has been bothering me. The last time I was Burt's primary doctor during daylight hours, he was on ventilator settings identical to the current settings. I am getting concerned that we haven't been able to improve his condition. Our running diagnosis is acute respiratory distress syndrome (ARDS) since the hemorrhage, but if his lung problems all stemmed from that, wouldn't they be improving by now? Was it time to explore other diagnoses?

The attending, who just rotated onto the ICU, is not so sure. "ARDS takes a long time to resolve," he says. "How long has it been?" Now it's my turn to be unsure, as I have not been here every day. No resident on our team has. I look at my paper to get the exact number of days right. We are all trying to piece together a story we didn't personally watch unfold, with large chunks of time blacked out from each of our vantage points.

I venture alternative diagnoses. "The blood clots in his legs make me worry about a PE"—a pulmonary embolism—"but he's been on prophylactic heparin, so it's less likely," I say. "We stopped that when his hemoglobin dropped, I think," a different resident points out. She was on call that day and placed the order, so she would know. "What day was that?" A third resident runs through the electronic chart, trying to track down the answer. We see orders for heparin started and stopped at various time points over Burt's ICU stay, a different doctor's name populating each order.

This is the reality of twenty-eight-hour shifts. Every day a different doctor flipped through notes on complex patients she couldn't know well. Huge lapses occurred: one resident didn't realize that in her post-call absence her patient from the day before was now intubated. Another casually started presenting the case of an empty room, missing that his former patient had been discharged. Someone always caught our mistakes, but this was our norm: we relied on the charts, played catchup, and tried to assemble bits of knowledge into coherent stories. We missed things. We also repeated things, once having an entire *Groundhog Day*–type discussion of whether a patient had heparin-induced thrombocytopenia because the doctors changed and the one who ordered the initial tests was off. We started heparin, stopped heparin; broadened antibiotics, narrowed antibiotics; trended hemoglobin, ignored hemoglobin.

Our lives were filled with "hey, before you sleep" texts to one another asking for clarification. During the day, we passed the Batphone back and forth. When it rang and we didn't have the answers, we tried to find the doctor who might.

"Hold on a second."

"Let me see if she's around."

"I don't know, but I can look in the chart."

One day, as I handed the Batphone to another resident, she slumped against the nurses' station and shook her first.

"No one knows anything about these patients," she said.

"It's chaos," I commiserated.

We were a revolving door of doctors, each with authority for one day and one night—and gone the next. Our schedules forced us to trade continuity over days for continuity over hours, with little regard for how this fragmented the big picture.

Burt's wife, Patricia, adapted to our rotating crew and developed her own tactics to deal with it. "You today?" she would ask. She learned to repeat the important stuff over and over, knowing it was impossible for us to communicate everything to one another.

The staunchest defenders of these hours denounce handoffs (that is, one doctor conferring, or "handing off," primary responsibility for their patients to another doctor) as a major argument against shorter shifts. Handing off patients allows details to slip between doctors, they say. But these arguments ignore an obvious fact: there is no way around handoffs. As long as doctors have to sleep, eat, and use the bathroom (not to mention live their lives), at some point there will be a break in care. Twenty-eight-hour calls do not eliminate handoffs; rather, they break the continuity of patients' care between doctors through choppy scheduling that treats doctors as interchangeable from day to day. These arguments miss the fact that it's not a win to pass off a patient at twenty-eight hours to a doctor who doesn't know the patient well compared to handing off at twelve or sixteen hours to a doctor who does.

Good medicine involves clear roles. While leading an emergency medical response, for example, I learned to say, "Ellen, please push 300 milligrams of amiodarone," instead of " 'Someone' push 300 milligrams of amiodarone." What twenty-eight-hour shifts create is a perpetual mindset of "I'm just covering today"—and "just coverage" doesn't allow for clear roles.

Good medicine means realizing when to step back, rearrange the picture, and change course; coverage dances around big decisions. Good medicine plans ahead for a meaningful recovery; coverage is keeping your patients unscathed until your shift ends. Good medicine means accountability; coverage diffuses it. We were so focused on putting one foot in front of the other that larger narratives, like whether Burt's respiratory failure should be improving by now, escaped us.

Twenty-eight-hour calls operate on the faulty assumption that doctors are interchangeable from one day to the next. They ignore the value that comes from building relationships and the insights that develop from seeing the story play out every day. In this setup we did the immediate work of responding to medical complications but struggled with anything longer term. Complexity? No one could think about it. Uncertainty? No one had enough context. Planning ahead? It was no one's job.

THE TWISTED BACKSTORY behind twenty-eight-hour calls is that they're actually an improvement. The old guard of medical culture says we earn our stripes as doctors partly by how grueling it is to become one. During our first few years as doctors, we are called "residents," a term that originated in the nineteenth century from the fact that these physicians often physically lived—or "resided"—in the hospital. While this is no longer exactly the case, residents still spend exorbitant amounts of time there.

And yet some doctors with this older mindset scoff at the softness of our current setup. You're complaining about 28-hour shifts? *We* used to do 48. You think 80-hour weeks are long? Try 120.

You learn to be a doctor through complete immersion. Some of this is necessary. You learn to be good by seeing enough patients to know the range of normal and abnormal and by being the point person grappling with hard choices. You remember what you did well and what could have been better. Did you miss a diagnosis? Try again. Are you unable to thread a central line? Try again. Did you say something wrong while sharing bad news? Try again. There is no shortage of agains in residency. I deeply valued that process of betterment—and feeling the evolution from fear to competency to excellence.

But left unchecked, this attitude can send doctors-in-training—and their patients—into dangerous territory. Decades of research from within the medical community have made an effort to downplay this fact. For most of history, doctors existed in their own world, meaning they regulated their own world. The alarm bells first rang in 1971, when three doctors published a paper in the *New England Journal of Medicine* showing that sleep-deprived first-year residents, otherwise known as interns, couldn't read ECGs as well as rested ones. Not only did the tired doctors miss critical arrhythmias, their moods were deeply affected, with exhausted interns feeling sadder and being harder on themselves.

Still, it was up to doctors to decide if this mattered, and most had no interest in reckoning with this knowledge. Unfortunately, it was a tragedy that drew national attention.

In 1984 Libby Zion was just eighteen years old, a freshman at Bennington College in Vermont. She was taking a prescribed medication called phenelzine for depression, and she was admitted to a hospital in New York for flu-like symptoms and spasmodic movements whose cause was not immediately clear. The two residents who admitted her discussed her case with Zion's regular family physician. They agreed to give IV fluids and observe. But shortly after, Zion became more agitated, and the residents prescribed the drug meperidine, or Demerol, and restrained her. Her temperature then climbed to 107 degrees, and as the resident physicians took measures to lower it, she suffered a cardiac arrest and died. Later, the cause was believed to be serotonin syndrome, caused by an interaction between the phenelzine she was taking at home and the meperidine she was prescribed in the hospital.

There are many gaps we can now identify to explain this tragic outcome. Impressively, the two residents in the hospital consulted with Zion's regular doctor and got a correct home medication list— something that easily could have fallen through the cracks opened by unshared medical records. Today the electronic charts would have notified a doctor of the drug interaction between meperidine and phenelzine, but the doctors in the 1980s didn't have that check. Zion's parents focused on another gap: they were convinced their daughter's death was due to overworked residents. They attributed the mental lapse in overlooking the drug-drug interaction to exhaustion and sleep deprivation from working extremely long shifts. Her father wrote an op-ed that splayed across the pages of the New York Times: "You don't need kindergarten to know that a resident working a 36-hour shift is in no condition to make any kind of judgment call—forget about life-and-death."

In 1989 New York State passed the "Libby Zion Law," which prohibited residents from working more than eighty hours a week or more than twenty-four consecutive hours. Many other states adopted similar limits.

Still, it took fourteen years for the ACGME, the organization in charge of residency hours at the national level, to adopt serious changes. In 2003 it too created similar regulations for all accredited medical training institutions in the United States. New standards limited residents to eighty hours per week averaged over four weeks and limited the length of individual shifts to thirty hours.

Maybe you should read that sentence again. Remarkably, shifts that were thirty consecutive hours long arose from a policy that *cut* hours.

In 2008 the National Academy of Medicine (then named the Institute of Medicine) upped the ante when it recommended that residents work no more than sixteen consecutive hours without sleep. The ACGME partially acted on this recommendation in 2011, prohibiting shifts exceeding sixteen consecutive hours for first-year residents.

Many celebrated what felt like long-overdue changes, but it's worth pausing to emphasize the fine print. These protections only applied to the first year of residency. Those considered more experienced residents—meaning second-year doctors and beyond—were immune to the new rules. It was as though getting promoted to your second year as a doctor canceled out the concerning science connecting sleep deprivation to impaired decision-making.

Even that concession was too much for some, with the announcement provoking a quick backlash that interns were being coddled. Doctors who disagreed with the new rules prosecuted their case in the language they knew best: large studies and small p-values to demonstrate statistical significance. They used data from Medicare and Veterans Affairs to scour millions of hospitalizations and pointed out no difference in important patient safety outcomes following the 2003 reductions in hours. Other studies associated the new rules in both 2003 and 2011 with less direct patient contact, more handoffs, decreased educational opportunities, and only minimally increased sleep.

So in 2017 the ACGME changed their stance, eliminating the sixteen-hour maximum for first-year doctors. Today, shifts of up to twenty-eight consecutive hours are fair game for all resident physicians. The ACGME press release stated a cap of twenty-four hours, a number that was widely quoted in the media. However, the fine print noted "plus up to four hours to manage necessary care transitions"—meaning, in practicality, twenty-eight hours. The ACGME defended the rule change with the language of scientific research. "The Task Force's decision on clinical experience and education hours was evidence-based," they assured the community. They cited a "preponderance of evidence" to support the idea that very long shifts are safe for patients and, again, facilitate "continuity of care," and that shorter shifts could hurt young doctors' professional development.

One piece of this "preponderance of evidence" was the Flexibility in Duty Hour Requirements for Surgical Trainees (FIRST) trial, in which first-year surgical residents were randomly assigned to max out at sixteen hours compared to twenty-eight hours. When the results were tallied, the trial found no differences in patient deaths or serious surgical complications between the groups.

This study of first-year surgeons was swiftly extrapolated to all doctors. However, conflating medical specialties is self-evidently problematic. Some resident surgeons argue they didn't want to scrub out in the middle of a case, as many surgical cases *do* run longer than sixteen hours. But for internal medicine doctors like me, there was no case to scrub out of. The argument in my specialty was that longer hours were better because we got to see our cases evolve, through their ups and downs, hour by hour. But of course my patients could medically crash at 2:00 a.m. or 9:00 a.m. When working sixteen-hour shifts, I oversaw plenty of patient cases as they evolved; then I went home to sleep, came back in the morning, and saw them evolve some more. There was nothing magical about twenty-eight hours.

A sensible person might take a step back and wonder if scientific trials are even the right way to decide workplace hours—for surgeons, internal medicine doctors, or anyone else. Many things in life don't need a randomized trial to reach a decision. My favorite example of this point was a parody published in the *British Medical Journal* that mockingly used a double-blind, randomized, placebo-controlled, crossover trial (hitting all of medicine's favorite buzz-words describing trial designs) to determine whether parachutes are successful interventions when jumping out of planes. The insinuation was that our obsession with evidence in medicine has led us to distort questions of common sense and human decency. It would be perfectly easy to design studies testing whether week-ends or no weekends are harmful for coal miners. I am sure if we dove deep enough into the data we could find differences in some outcomes and no differences in others. But would we?

We would never design the coal-miner study because we appre-ciate that basic workplace rights should not be contingent on the results of an experiment. We understand that these rights are ques-tions not of science but of humanity.

Medicine, however, promised more data—more data on pin-pointing the exact number of hours that would break us, wrapped up in the shiny language of a randomized clinical trial; more data on whether patients were harmed, topped with a bow of statistical significance. To prove that the FIRST trial could be extrapolated to internal medicine residents, the Individualized Comparative Effectiveness of Models Optimizing Patient Safety and Resident Education (iCOMPARE) trial—funded by the National Heart, Lung, and Blood Institute and the ACGME and led by investi-gators at Johns Hopkins University School of Medicine and the University of Pennsylvania—experimented on thousands more residents at sixty-three hospitals across the country.

I was one of those residents. A few months before the trial launched, I was in my last year of medical school and flying around the country interviewing at different hospitals for residency. Along the trail, I came across hospital after hospital that boasted of their involvement in the trial. "We are proudly participating in iCOM-PARE next year," they would say.

And by "we," they really meant "you."

The trial raised ethical red flags for me. Before I entered medicine, I interned at a bioethics advisory panel in Washington, DC, studying informed consent in research conducted on human subjects. Now I was going to be a subject in a study I did not directly consent to, examining whether warping my sense of time would affect whether I harmed patients. I wondered how this was ethical. I wondered how hospital residency directors—but not actual residents, much less patients—signing on the dotted line amounted to true informed consent. And on a personal level, I resented being conscripted into something that was not at all an academic exercise but would deeply affect my life and my ability to care for patients. But I needed to go to residency. I kept my concerns to myself, grumbled only to close family and friends, and thanked every hospital for their consideration.

I later learned I wasn't alone. In 2015 a different think tank called Public Citizen and the American Medical Student Association called both the FIRST and iCOMPARE trials "highly unethical" and asked for an investigation from the Office for Human Research Protections. Even after multiple requests, the office took no action, prompting Public Citizen to call them a "culpable party in this unethical research." The iCOMPARE trial protocol claimed that the research carried "no more than minimal risk," allowing them to waive getting informed consent. As an additional justification, they invoked the scale of the research, asserting it would not be feasible to obtain consent from the thousands of patients who would be involved. Some hospitals' Institutional Review Board applications stated that the hospitals were not involved in human research because the residency programs themselves were the research subjects. It was kind of like saying people didn't have to consent because the building consented.

Half the participating hospitals would have their first-year residents work twenty-eight-hour shifts while the other half retained sixteen-hour caps. To my great relief, the coin flip landed me in the sixteen-hour group. (Again, however, I was only shielded from twenty-eight-hour shifts for one year.) A few years later, I read with interest the published results of the experiment. Much like the FIRST trial, iCOMPARE showed that no more patients died when their doctors worked for twenty-eight hours straight compared to sixteen hours. Proponents of twenty-eight-hour calls cheered, buoyed by outcomes that supported their gut instincts. Opponents parsed the study, pointing out that patient death is an extraordinarily low bar for measuring outcomes.

Indeed, the study did not attempt to detect the flaws of fragmentation I experienced with Burt and my other ICU patients. Glaring patient safety failures, such as an accidental laceration, were flagged, but the study did not examine details such as time on a ventilator that necessitated a tracheostomy caused by confusing handoffs. It probed no questions of whether patients lingered in critical care limbo because of a chronic coverage mentality that diffused responsibility for helping them recover. It didn't capture the labor of frantic text exchanges or the impact that repeating interventions had on our patients' quality of life as we played catchup. It didn't look at the burden patients experienced from repeating information to new doctors daily or the confusion stemming from not having a go-to primary doctor.

The study did show that doctors' well-being suffered the more consecutive hours they worked. Additionally, doctors said their education was worse with the longer hours. Although all this was demonstrated in medicine's favorite language—statistical significance—these results were brushed off. The conclusion that no patients were massacred was apparently enough to grant hospitals permission to continue these shifts.

Even aside from the questionable ethics involved, one could also query the design of these studies. They were designed to prove (or disprove) the hypothesis that twenty-eight-hour calls were no less safe than regular hours: not that twenty-eight-hour calls were *better* in any way, just that they weren't a lot worse. Even if the result is "positive"—meaning no major differences in patient safety were found—should that convince anybody that twenty-eight-hour shifts are the way to go? The researchers could just as easily have designed a study with the inverse hypothesis, asking if sixteen-hour shifts were no worse than twenty-eight-hour shifts. In that case, the very same "positive" result—no differences in patient deaths—could be used to justify the shorter shifts. That they didn't design the study to ask that question is suggestive of their motivations.

The premise of these trials is so distorted to reflect the opinion that longer hours are favorable that one might have to read them several times just to figure out who's who. The doctors working twenty-eight-hour shifts are in the nice-sounding "flexible" group. Another positive label they carry is "less restrictive."

I asked the ACGME how longer hours foster continuity of care, and they responded by email. As of 2022, they said there were no further planned or proposed changes to existing work hours. They cited an editorial accompanying the iCOMPARE trial in which two physicians at Brigham and Women's Hospital at Harvard Medical School wrote, "We can confidently say that working flexible hours, still within the 80-hour constraints, does not result in higher patient mortality than working standard hours." As a result, "the issue of duty hours can now, in many ways, be laid to rest," the ACGME summarized their perspective.

And so nearly forty years after the tragic death of Libby Zion and her father's impassioned call to action, little has changed. Every so often, doctors and other concerned citizens will publish articles tearing apart twenty-eight-hour calls. But they are shouting into broken megaphones to the ones setting the schedules.

RESIDENTS AND FELLOWS ARE DOCTORS. During my six years in these positions, whether I worked regular shifts, overnight shifts, or twenty-eight-hour calls, I was the doctor responsible for life-and-death decisions about extraordinarily sick and complex patients. I admitted patients and managed them and did all the on-the-ground work of medical care. But what makes resident and fellow doctors unique is that they always have a degree of supervision from an attending physician they can call if they need help. Doing a residency is required to become a fully licensed, independently practicing physician in this country.

For patients like Burt Klein whose lives are in these doctors' hands, it makes little difference what exactly they are called. But the mysterious middle ground between independent physician and physician-in-training is important because it's what allows twenty-eight-hour shifts to persist.

Doctors are assigned to residency by the "Match," an algorithm that pairs graduating medical students with hospitals based on their ranked preferences. The Match was fueled by an admirable goal: getting as many graduating medical students into residency spots as possible. The algorithm's designer, Alvin Roth, was even awarded a Nobel Prize in Economics. But the fallout of a hiring system that pairs doctors with a single place of employment is one that strips them of any negotiating power. That means hospitals have mostly free rein to keep residents' hours high and pay low. Without central oversight, it's up to individual hospital leaders to decide how to structure residents' work hours. Good leadership certainly exists; some set humane schedules and give well-deserved thought to how to optimize the Jenga of patient care, resident education, and employee well-being.

But we cannot ignore what this system enables: hospitals taking advantage of resident physicians as the cheapest available skilled labor. Hour by hour, resident physicians generally earn around a minimum wage, which can make them the lowest-paid employees in a hospital. Nurse practitioners and physician assistants make about twice the salary of resident physicians, while residents work hours twice as long. Hiring an attending physician, nurse practitioner, or physician assistant to do the work of a resident would cost hospitals more. So a financial strategy can be to work residents and fellows longer and harder.

In 2002 a group of resident physicians brought a class-action lawsuit against the ACGME, the Association of American Medical Colleges (AAMC), and twenty-seven teaching hospitals, claiming that the Match violated antitrust laws. By removing competition, the lawsuit alleged, the Match suppressed residents' salaries to an artificial low. A federal district court initially ruled that the Match might be an illegal restraint on trade. But after intense lobbying from the AAMC and American Hospital Association, Congress quickly enacted legislation declaring medical training programs exempt. The lawsuit was thrown out of court.

It is notable that in this drought of choice, twenty-eight-hour shifts continue to be framed as a choice. "It is important to note that 24 hours is a ceiling, not a floor," the 2017 ACGME press release said. "Residents in many specialties may never experience a 24-hour clinical work period." In the *New York Times*, Stephen Evans, the chair of the American Board of Surgery and chief medical officer for MedStar Health, was quoted: "If you are a pediatric first-year resident taking care of a critically ill patient, and the child dies, do you just walk away from the family because the 16 hours are up?"

"Wouldn't you want to stay for your patient?" is a convenient argument, repeated ad nauseam, because it capitalizes on doctors' moral compasses while having nothing to do with the situation at hand. I and every other doctor I know has gladly stayed late for a patient in need. But there is a difference between choosing to stay for your patient when the situation calls for it and being obligated to work lengthy shifts on a regular basis. Once twenty-eight-hour shifts are considered fair game, these hours aren't merely permitted when an individual doctor believes it is best for her patient or her learning. Instead, schedules are constructed with these hours as their backbone for the doctors lowest on the food chain. They become mandated shifts that entail all the work a hospital shift requires—whether that's providing continuity with existing patients or caring for new ones. As it happens, the continuity between a doctor and a patient that's endlessly used to defend these shifts in theory is completely erased in practice. Under the guise of combating fragmentation, extremely long shifts are a root cause in aggravating it.

FIXING THIS IS MADDENINGLY SIMPLE. During my last year of residency, one of my colleagues proposed changing twenty-eight-hour shifts to shifts of twelve hours in the medical ICU. Interestingly, my discussions with my co-residents at the time didn't fixate on anything related to our emotions or exhaustion. Instead, our arguments—for or against—revolved mostly around continuity of patient care. I learned that many others had the same revelation I experienced while caring for Burt: that longer hours actually break up continuity with patients. We swapped stories about losing sight of the bigger picture as overtired physicians received continuity in hours in lieu of a more impactful continuity we would get from overseeing the same patients from day to day.

Burt Klein didn't suffer the same fate as Libby Zion, but I'm sobered to think of the extra efforts required to compensate for our schedule-induced lapses. The note about his possibly misplaced feeding tube I had tucked away became relevant again one day—which happened to be my day off sleeping—when his bedside nurse astutely noted distension in his abdomen. The steroids that were meant to treat his lungs had weakened his gut to the point of perforation, causing tube feeds to spill out into his abdominal cavity. It took some extra time, many texts exchanged from home, and scrambling, but we took care of it. Despite a lot of false starts and halting medications, his lungs slowly recovered. So did his kidneys and his platelet levels.

I thought of Burt when our residency reform committee weighed in on my colleague's proposal. The vote was in support of regular shifts. So the next time I rotated through the ICU, instead of working twenty-eight consecutive hours, I worked consistent twelve-hours shifts. That meant the same doctors had ownership over the same patients every day (and every night).

If this was an experiment, I was my own control. In an instant, I said goodbye to staggered caffeine shots and five-minute naps. Our clandestine network of slipping one another Coke Zeroes and covering the Batphone to allow daytime naps evaporated.

That wasn't all that changed. Our handoffs were smoother because we all knew the patients better. Our relationships with nurses improved, as communication lines opened and nurses no longer had to do their own internal calculus as to whether something was worth waking the doctor. My own patient care was unquestionably more thoughtful, more holistic, and more detail oriented. It wasn't just because I was well rested. My accountability was different. I was no longer trying to keep a list of patients stable until my shift ended. Every day I pushed bit by bit toward my patients' larger recoveries, which I was now able to envision clearly.

The medical community has a choice. We can continue to have the same debate for five more decades. We can pour money into bigger studies, get in the weeds of research design, and wax poetic about tiny differences in outcomes. We can experiment on thousands more doctors who just want to do their jobs and who never agreed to be guinea pigs.

Or we can end this right now.

This doesn't have to take decades. It won't take wrangling multibillion-dollar software companies or wading through the partisan fights of policy change. If we're looking for the low-hanging fruit of fragmentation in medicine, twenty-eight-hour shifts are moldy apples on the ground. What it takes to clean them up is a decision: We do have enough evidence to regulate doctors' consecutive hours. More important, we have enough humanity to do so.

Imagine it's the person you love most who has fallen critically ill. Behind door number one is the doctor on hour twenty-three out of twenty-eight. Behind door number two is the doctor who is there every day, working twelve hours at a time. Who would you choose?

Chapter 6

Reinventing Primary Care

E VENTUALLY, BURT LEFT THE HOSPITAL. WHAT HE NEEDED next was what Jin Wong needed: "someone" who could see him on a regular basis and guide him toward recovery.

These were the thoughts running through my mind at the end of a decade of medical training. After four years of medical school, three as a resident, and three as a fellow, I was fully trained to practice internal medicine, oncology, and hematology. It was time to find an attending job. As I searched, I thought seriously about where I wanted to work and the patients I wanted to see: mostly sick patients in the hospital or mostly outpatients in the clinic? Should I stay broad, seeing patients with all kinds of cancer or focus on one or two types?

But even as I pondered patients and pathologies, I remained inescapably aware of the harms created by our fragmented systems and how I could best position myself within them to do good. For me a satisfying job had to include follow-up: I wanted to care for the whole patient over time.

The most straightforward path for someone with my training would have been to join an oncology practice. But that prospect still featured gaps in care. I had witnessed a version of the same story many times: when a patient with cancer develops a new problem, where does he turn? Imagine a person with lymphoma and on chemotherapy develops a red, painful knee. He calls his oncologist, who says it's not from the chemotherapy and recommends he ask his primary care doctor. The primary care doctor diagnoses gout but is unsure whether prescribing a gout medication could interfere with the cancer treatment and suggests he ask his oncologist.

This is not a rare story. As of 2019, there were an estimated 16.9 million cancer survivors in the United States; that number is projected to reach 26.1 million by 2040. As I dove into the literature to understand the gaps in care for patients with cancer, one quote stopped me in my tracks: "Internists do not understand my cancer and oncologists do not understand my non-cancer health maintenance needs, such as monitoring cholesterol and blood pressure," a patient said. Even those who are cured of their cancer may experience a host of new problems: osteoporosis, infertility, premature menopause, heart disease, memory problems, nerve damage, risk of second cancers, fatigue, and depression. With no one tasked to address them, these needs often go unmet.

Seeing my patients struggle to navigate this world, I realized I was in a position where I could actually do something about it. But how?

I reached out to anyone I thought could help. I discovered a primary care doctor and an oncologist in a community practice ninety miles north of me who teamed up to provide ninety-minute visits with patients who had recently finished cancer treatment. I spoke to an oncologist in Southern California who spent one day a week seeing complex cancer survivors in one- to two-hour visits. Some suggested I carve out cancer survivorship as a subspecialty, where I could be the doctor who bridged care between the oncologist and the primary care doctor. But combating fragmentation meant I wanted to consolidate my patients' care; I worried adding a third doctor to the mix could complicate it.

Finally, I had an epiphany: the answer lay not in oncology but in primary care. I wanted to create a primary care practice that provided comprehensive care for cancer patients. A primary care doctor is the "someone" so many patients need. A primary care doctor manages long-term symptoms and chronic diseases. A primary care doctor prevents. A primary care doctor takes care of the entire patient over time. A primary care doctor is the quarterback. A primary doctor can detangle and safeguard the patient's full story.

I drew inspiration from the fact that primary care targeted to a specific population was not a new idea. Geriatrics is primary care with a special focus on older adults. A general pediatrician is a primary care doctor for younger patients. My idea was primary care with a special focus on patients with cancer, anywhere along the spectrum—from surviving a stage 1 breast cancer twenty years ago to living with metastatic lung cancer today. My vision was to channel my expertise in both internal medicine and oncology to address all my patients' medical needs—cancer related and otherwise—in one place.

With the support of a primary care doctor at Stanford Medicine who had piloted visits for cancer survivors, I pitched the idea to my institution. Amazingly, their biggest concern was not whether my idea would work but whether I would be happy doing it. Knowing I had gone through a rigorous oncology and hematology fellowship during which I saw patients through modern miracles of immunotherapy and bone marrow transplants, one interviewer asked, "Are you sure you want to treat back pain and hypertension?" I said yes because that's where the need was.

But my interviewer's surprise at my pivot in specialty was not surprising. The realizations I personally reached about primary care as the key to combating fragmentation fly in the face of a reality in which primary care has been systemically undervalued and a crisis has been building for decades. National spending on primary care constitutes a mere 5 to 7 percent of all health care spending. Primary care physicians are among the lowest-paid doctors, earning half the salaries of some specialists who do procedures, such as orthopedists and plastic surgeons. Fewer graduating medical students are choosing the field. Even more concerning is a growing burnout crisis, leading fully established and highly trained primary care doctors to quit in droves. Data published by the Association of American Medical Colleges predict a shortage of 17,800 to 48,000 primary care physicians by 2034. Even people who have primary care doctors struggle to access them, plagued by inconvenient scheduling, antiquated methods of communication, and appointment shortages.

What is going on?

These disconnects underscore the gravity of what's at stake. Just as the electronic charts hold the promise to connect health data seamlessly if done well but can deepen existing fractures when designed poorly, how we design primary care in this nation has the power to solve or exacerbate fragmented follow-up. If we get it right, primary care can narrow the ever-growing chasm of patients who need regular, consistent, long-term medical care. But when it's poorly designed, primary care becomes yet another casualty of America's fragmented health care system, flattening relationships that can accomplish so much into sporadic transactions that do so little.

As I imagined my own practice, I became consumed by the questions: what would ideal primary care look like, and how would that differ from what we have now?

A DOCTOR NAMED MONIQUE TELLO embodies what we have now. For thirteen years, Tello worked as a primary care doctor at Massachusetts General Hospital in Boston. She had accrued a practice of about a thousand patients, most of them women. Nobody, especially not her past self, could have anticipated her next career move.

She quit.

"The administrative burden tipped me over the edge," she told me over the phone. Tello appreciated the move to electronic charts. An early adopter of her hospital's system, Epic, she had even become a "Super User" who taught other providers. But Epic's existence became a conduit for her workload to spill into all hours of the day. "It was like an eternal game of Whac-A-Mole: no matter how hard you worked at it or how much time you spent, that InBasket would just fill right up again."

The "InBasket" is the secure inbox of Epic's electronic charts. It is where we respond to patient questions, review test results, refill prescriptions, coordinate with other providers, and sign notes. Tello worked part time, seeing patients two and a half days per week. A scribe who listened in to her visits remotely transcribed her notes. But even with these layers of support, "I was never able to grasp how there was so much work in the off hours," she said.

The situation came to a head during a vacation. In 2021 she traveled to Guatemala to visit family she hadn't seen in two years because of the coronavirus pandemic. Every day for a week, she logged into the charts remotely to deal with tasks. Sometimes they were urgent, such as a patient's messaging about symptoms of a urinary tract infection that would require her to prescribe antibiotics.

It wasn't until she got back that Tello took serious stock of what happened. She returned to Boston on a Saturday. When she logged back in on Sunday and still had more to do, the realization struck. "This is insane," she remembered thinking. "I just spent my vacation touching the [electronic health record] every day, and I'm still not caught up." It hit her then: "I will never be caught up." And her next thought was, "I can't keep doing this."

She began reaching out to friends who had found jobs outside of traditional medicine. It dawned on her that there was a world of other options where she could use her medical knowledge and receive adequate support at the same time. "I was really struck hearing the same story over and over," she said of her colleagues who left medicine for industry. "It was like, now I have support. I have resources. I can actually contribute the way I want to contribute."

She found a job at a biotechnology company, gave her clinic three months' notice, and told her patients goodbye.

I met Tello through a Facebook group of doctors helping doctors find alternative careers. Some of the posts gave me a feeling of attending an Alcoholics Anonymous meeting. Doctors were praised for working up the courage to admit their lives weren't working out. They knew things were bad but worried getting out could be worse. They feared hurting their families. They felt ashamed of going into debt. Meanwhile, the group consistently responded with kindness, validation, and support. They shared ideas: there were doctors who developed successful second careers in research, insurance claim review, drug development, web design, and even real estate.

In addition to Tello, I connected by phone with a few other primary care doctors. Their stories were similar: visits were getting shorter, and the workload was growing. They spent more time on clerical tasks than meaningful care, and the electronic charts only amplified the imbalance. They felt like cogs in a machine, with their workflows controlled by administrators who didn't understand what either doctors or patients need. Dana Corriel, who left primary care after about fifteen years in practice and founded a digital branding company for doctors, described it this way: "You're a factory worker. You can be a nine-to-five factory worker, and that's fine. But if you want me to be the doctor I trained for that truly cares and bends over backwards to see my patients healthy, I shouldn't be a factory worker. I should be in charge."

IN THE FALL OF 2021—despite warnings of burnout and general consternation from some of my colleagues—I opened my primary care clinic. Word got around, and quickly I was booked. About half of my patients are cancer survivors and those at high risk: I am the primary doctor for childhood cancer survivors who have now reached adulthood, patients with genetic syndromes conferring increased cancer risks, adults with active cancer, and adult cancer survivors many years out. So many patients have expressed to me they are stunned that my clinic exists. It has been one of my greatest privileges to create one solution to the gaps I watched my patients battle firsthand.

The other half of my practice is standard primary care in all its diversity. Doing this work, I now believe more than ever that primary care is the answer to knitting together the fragmented relationships between patients and doctors. Seeing patients over time allows me to develop relationships and establish trust. Being the point person lets me consolidate recommendations from specialists and help my patients prioritize next steps. Above all else, that remarkable ability to recommend something new—and then "see you next month"—allows us to make incremental improvements together.

Yet when I opened my practice, it also didn't take long for me to internalize the assembly-line economics Corriel and the others were talking about. Though the concept of my clinic was novel, I set up shop within a traditional health care organization, paid for by traditional methods of reimbursement. My days were packed with patient appointments from 8:00 a.m. to 5:00 p.m., back-to-back in thirty-minute slots. As word about my new clinic spread and my schedule quickly filled, I just as swiftly grappled with a question: when was I supposed to do all the *other* work of patient care?

Recently I met a twenty-six-year-old who came to see me as his new doctor. He had been diagnosed with leukemia at age fourteen and treated with two years of chemotherapy and a bone marrow transplant. After the transplant, he had developed graft-versus-host disease, a serious condition where the new bone marrow recognizes the patient's own body as foreign and attacks it. It left him with a blistering skin rash and intestinal damage. Then the years of steroids he was given to quell his immune system caused necrosis of his hip bone, and he underwent a total hip replacement. Now he struggled to make his way back into anything that resembled a normal life. He continued to live in his childhood bedroom. He suffered from insomnia to the point that his sleep schedule was almost completely reversed.

In the clinic room, we talked through it all. He told me about the anxiety that accompanied walking into any doctor's office, including mine. His skin still itched, and his eyes felt gritty. He had put on twenty pounds because his hip ached when he tried to exercise. I set expectations about which symptoms we could potentially improve and which might involve adjusting to a new normal. I reviewed all the cancer treatments he had received and recommended tests for monitoring health problems that can crop up later: an echocardiogram of his heart, tests of his lung function, and blood draws to evaluate hormones. Later, as I wrote a note in his chart, I noticed in a separate electronic tab that his pediatric oncologist had recently done hormone tests that returned abnormal results. A subsequent brain MRI showed what looked like a mass in his pituitary gland. I froze. I tried to follow the thread through dozens of clicks. I gathered that he had lost insurance during his transition to adulthood. No doctor even followed up on the mass. I messaged an endocrine specialist, asking her to review the MRI. Then I sent the patient a message with this new information we had skipped during the visit.

All of this took time: time to dig through his electronic chart, map out a monitoring plan, write a note, message other doctors, research rare pituitary tumors, and circle back and contact the patient. Yet the only time that payers compensated for treating this patient was our thirty-minute visit, which I spent face to face with him. And I am lucky: it is common for a primary care doctor to get just fifteen minutes per patient to do all this work.

In my estimate, up to half of a primary care doctor's work happens outside the patient room. None of this is directly paid for. How can this be?

As of 2021, 88 percent of medical care in the nation operates according to a payment model called fee-for-service. The basics of this model go as far back as Hammurabi. According to the rates inscribed on clay tablets in the eighteenth century B.C., if a physician set a broken bone, the patient paid five shekels of silver (two shekels if the patient was a slave). If a physician made a deep incision with a lancet of bronze, the cost was ten shekels.

This was fine in Hammurabi's day, when there was no such thing as living with chronic illness and a doctor's choices were limited. But today this means most clinics can bill only for what is considered a medical service: an operation, a round of chemotherapy, a joint injection. For primary care doctors, that medical service has been commodified into the office visit. Nothing else counts: not written messages between patients and doctors; not discussion between doctors and other doctors; not communication between patients and other team members such as medical assistants; until 2020, not phone calls (this changed only because of Covid); not obtaining and reviewing charts or writing notes outside the time billed for the visit. It is as if a tenured university professor were paid only for back-to-back lectures in the classroom, with the time spent preparing the course material, creating syllabi and problem sets, grading exams, answering student questions, and doing her own research considered irrelevant.

In 2010 the Affordable Care Act tried to incentivize doctors' offices away from fee-for-service toward more holistic payment models. One way it did this was by allowing health care organizations with at least five thousand patients on Medicare to contract with the government and receive up to 60 percent of cost savings. But the dominant payment models nationwide have been slow to change. Some clinics have tried to improve the situation by paying individual doctors a fixed salary to avoid creating individual incentives to overbook and overtreat (this is my situation, and I'm relieved that's the case). However, with most *organizations* still receiving funding from fee-for-service, even doctors who get paid a fixed salary become trapped in the factory Corriel described: administrators push primary care doctors into doing more on the assembly line. This is why the average primary care doctor sees twenty to twenty-five patients a day, in fifteen-minute slots, with their total practices consisting of over two thousand patients.

All the while, the work is only growing. Primary care doctors spend more time interacting with electronic charts than any other outpatient specialty. Compared to surgeons, they receive more than twice as many messages from other staff, five times as many messages from patients, and fifteen times as many prescription messages every day. And, unlike specialists, primary care doctors generally lack adequate support staff to divvy up this work. The average primary care clinic agonizes over hiring another medical assistant while orthopedic surgeons down the hall enjoy state-of-the-art technologies and teams of highly trained coworkers. With no solution paid for, the party line to primary care doctors is to squeeze it in. Do it when you're off the clock. We don't know how, but just do it anyway.

The consequences are exactly as expected. Primary care—the very specialty that is supposed to be the most holistic—is fragmented into infrequent office visits, with doctors given no time to do any follow-up in between. Because a primary care doctor generally has over two thousand patients, each patient will struggle to access that doctor; so patients hoard a year's worth of problems for those coveted face-to-face slots. Meanwhile, doctors like me would love to adapt to modern channels of communication and engage in regular back and forth. Yet whenever test results on my patients come back as abnormal, I wrestle with whether to schedule another office visit with my patient to review them. I know another thirty minutes (plus travel time, if they come in person) out of *their* schedule is not ideal. But that's the only way I can allot any time for myself. Similarly, I struggle with whether to advise my patients to message me for ongoing issues: tell me how you are feeling on the new medication in one week; send me your blood pressure measurements. Making time for this uncompensated workload outside my scheduled workload means I chart notes at lunch. I shoot off messages in between seeing patients. Like Monique Tello, I drown in to-dos. Often I fall behind.

We have designed a system that puts patients' needs and doctors' ability to meet them fundamentally at odds. Astoundingly, primary care doctors are squeezing more and more work in, while patients are communicating with them less and less. As good doctors try to do it all anyway and burn out, many choose to go part time because everybody knows the secret: part time is actually full time. Others leave medicine completely. The medical establishment has responded to this crisis largely with an answer of "wellness." They arrange ice cream socials. They encourage doctors to meditate and do yoga. But many, including Tello, aren't buying it. "It's not about yoga, it's not about therapy, because it's not on us," she told me.

True wellness—for both doctors and patients—would address the underlying problems. Primary care doctors need more time caring for patients and working at the top of our licenses. Patients need convenient access to a regular doctor who knows them well. One way to get there is tinkering around the edges—hiring an extra medical assistant to triage messages or a scribe to write notes.

Or we can take a big step back and start from scratch.

"OUR TASK WAS TO DISRUPT THINGS," Alan Glaseroff, cofounder of Stanford Coordinated Care (SCC), told me in 2021. I first learned about SCC by happenstance. During my residency, I worked in a primary care clinic Tuesday and Thursday afternoons on the third floor of a building a few blocks from the hospital. On the fourth floor was a clinic I didn't know much about. I would see the bronze nameplate outside the elevators in the lobby, and once I skimmed an internal press release. But I didn't pay much attention until one day I was chatting with a colleague about innovative ways to do primary care. She suggested I look into SCC and connected me to the doctors by email.

I learned that it started with a puzzle: 5 percent of patients accounted for 50 percent of costs. In 2011 Arnold Milstein, the executive director of Stanford Medicine's Clinical Excellence Research Center, was looking at health expenditures for Stanford Medicine employees and their dependents and saw a small group driving up costs for the insurance plan. He called Glaseroff, a primary care doctor located about three hundred miles north in Humboldt County, and asked for his help in thinking up a way to provide better care for these patients. Glaseroff had gained a reputation for overseeing the Humboldt Diabetes Project, which had reduced the county death rate from diabetes by 29 percent between 2003 and 2008 compared to a 0 percent change in the state of California as a whole. Glaseroff then sought input from Ann Lindsay—a primary care physician, co-owner of his practice, public health officer for Humboldt County, and his wife. Lindsay had earned renown for eradicating an outbreak of shigellosis (an intestinal infection causing diarrhea) in a homeless encampment on a beach jetty. The couple made the long drive down to Palo Alto to see if they could help.

Glaseroff told me the first thing they did was hold "Skunk Works"—a brainstorming strategy that was originally developed in the weaponry and defense industries. Its name comes from a comic strip called *Li'l Abner* that depicted a mysterious place deep in the forest where a beverage was brewed from skunks, old shoes, and other strange ingredients—exuding an odor so hideous that everyone who worked there was left alone. You have to brainstorm new health care ideas in secret, Glaseroff explained. If you do it out in the open, bureaucracy will catch on to the stench and try to quash it.

Part of that brainstorming involved going straight to the source. Glaseroff and Lindsay interviewed hospitalized patients with chronic illnesses and asked them what they wanted out of their medical care. They learned that patients liked their doctors but felt the system was hard to use. They felt bombarded with facts when they needed to learn how to live with their illnesses. The best teachers were peers going through something similar. Many patients had childhood traumas that later contributed to behaviors that caused poor health. Glaseroff and Lindsay compiled the messages they heard most into seven core elements. Then they struck a deal with the patients: we will provide you primary care that addresses all of this, they promised. In return please call us before you decide to go to the emergency room, and let us know if you are hospitalized elsewhere.

To get the clinic up and running, Glaseroff and Lindsay knew that getting payment à la Hammurabi was a nonstarter. Instead, they asked for a lump sum upfront from Stanford University's insurance plan to invest in a medical team that could remain accessible and involved. They determined this number by looking at the patients who incurred the highest costs (on average they cost the insurance plan $43,000 each year) and dividing by the total cost of the providers they wanted to hire. The clinic would need $286 per patient each month from the insurance plan, they calculated. It was considered doable, and the insurance company agreed.

In 2012 the new clinic—Stanford Coordinated Care—opened. Its employees consisted of Glaseroff and Lindsay, a physical therapist, a nurse, a social worker, a pharmacist, a dietitian, and four care coordinators. The care coordinator job was most similar to that of a medical assistant, who in a typical practice is responsible for bringing patients in from the waiting room, taking vital signs, and restocking clean gowns. But the name change was intentional, signaling a corresponding change in responsibility. The care coordinator was "built as a peer role" for the patients, Glaseroff explained. For these positions, he and Lindsay recruited people certified as medical assistants and then spent a month training them to coach patients and stay present in the exam room, establishing themselves as familiar, credible messengers.

To qualify for the clinic, patients had to meet two intake criteria: they had to be employees of Stanford University or family members, and they had to have a chronic or complex medical condition. Most patients, as I would come to see, had multiple conditions.

By the time I visited in 2017, Glaseroff and Lindsay had returned home to Humboldt and passed the reins to the doctors Kathan Vollrath and Nancy Cuan. I climbed the four flights of stairs one Monday morning and looked for their office but couldn't find it. Instead, I entered a large team room, where staff desks with computer stations lined the four walls. I took a seat at a table in the center as the doctors welcomed me and introduced me to everyone else. Smiling faces spun to greet me as I met two care coordinators, a social worker, a dietitian, and an occupational therapist.

The day started with the group convening and reviewing a short list of patients who had active questions. One patient had intense anxiety around needles and asked for something to help him through a vaccine scheduled that morning. Another had developed severe abdominal pain and was on his way to a local emergency room. Already I was struck by what was happening: not only did everyone in the room participate; everyone *knew* these patients. No one said, "Hold on a second; let me pull up the chart."

After the urgent issues were addressed, the team split up to see patients. I glanced at the electronic chart of the first patient on the physician's schedule, a man I'll call John. His medical problems included high blood pressure, high cholesterol, obesity, chronic lower back pain, diabetes, anxiety, and panic attacks. He was well known to the clinic, and he came that day to address a few issues: a new headache, progress on his weight loss, and insomnia.

I entered the exam room with a care coordinator, who gathered the story: John's headache had been plaguing him for three days. The pain was a five out of ten. It came and went. It felt like a rubber band squeezing both temples. Tylenol helped a little.

We were in the room for about fifteen minutes. Then the doctor joined. She asked a lot of questions while the care coordinator sat at the computer typing notes. Why was this happening? "Sleep was bad lately," John said. Was it trouble falling asleep or staying asleep? The latter—he would awaken at 2:00 or 3:00 a.m. Had this happened before? Yes, when he was stressed. Was he stressed now? He was. How did he deal with stress before? Exercise. And now? He hadn't exercised as much. Why? Pain at the bottom of his right foot made it hurt to walk. He took off his shoes and socks. The doctor diagnosed him with plantar fasciitis and recommended fitted insoles for his sneakers. In the meantime, he had an exercise bike at home. Could he do that instead? "I think so." What was stopping him? "Nothing really," he admitted.

To break the current headache, the doctor recommended mild sleep aids to help reset his sleep-wake cycle. She prescribed the anti-inflammatory naproxen for pain. Finally, for the muscle tightness in John's neck, she recommended a special kind of exercise therapy called Feldenkrais. John thanked her. Then he simply walked into another room.

As I followed him, surreptitiously googling on my phone what Feldenkrais entailed (I discovered it's a gentle, mindful form of movement therapy), I thought about what would have happened had John visited my clinic one floor down. Here the visit with the doctor and care coordinator that diligently addressed each of his medical issues (and uncovered how they were related) took about an hour. Maybe I would have taken that hour too, but it would come at the cost of my next patients' time. I was unfortunately used to this. When I started out, my name and photo were projected on a screen in the waiting room, and on especially busy days I would watch the numbers add up under my face: Dr. Yurkiewicz, running fifteen minutes late, twenty minutes late, thirty minutes late.

Alternatively, I would have broken John's care into pieces: discuss headaches and sleep today; follow up to address foot pain and exercise. Arranging for him to see a physical therapist would have involved typing a referral into the computer, telling John he would get a callback, and having him schedule his appointment another day in another building. By that time, his head and neck pain could be long gone or way worse. To know how it went, I would have to check the chart, as I didn't directly communicate with the therapist. I would write the note myself, either knocking out something brief in the few minutes before seeing my next patient or writing something more detailed from home that evening.

At Stanford Coordinated Care, each visit with a new patient was scheduled for a whopping two hours. Patients coming for follow-up saw the doctor for an hour. "It was my dream type of appointment," Cuan told me later. Prior to joining the clinic, Cuan was beginning to feel burned out. She had been working as a primary care doctor in a county hospital for over fifteen years. In addition to seeing her own patients, she had a leadership and teaching role with residents. When she worked with two residents, 15-minute visits became 7.5-minute visits. "I felt I couldn't do justice to the patients or to teaching," she said.

Vollrath shared a similar story. On first learning about SCC, "I had this Oliver Twist feeling," she told me. "I was like a little street urchin looking in a window at the most luxurious feast you could ever imagine." She too had been a primary care doctor at a county hospital—a job that spoke to her because she wanted to provide excellent care for patients regardless of their ability to pay. But budget cuts after the 2008 recession left her at once pressured by administrators to squeeze in more patients on the assembly line while receiving fewer resources to help them. One day, after eighteen years at the county hospital and while her house was quiet, she found SCC through an internet search and sent out her résumé. "Alan [Glaseroff] was talking about things like hour-long appointments and medical systems that could do things," she told me. "I thought, 'This sounds crazy, but if it's real, I have to try.'"

There was something else during John's visit that caught my attention. He had high blood pressure, and in the clinic that day, his systolic blood pressure reached 190. Was the headache causing the high blood pressure, or was the high blood pressure causing the headache? I was pondering whether John was experiencing something called hypertensive emergency, a dangerous phenomenon where blood pressure shoots up so high that it damages organs. If John had called after hours, any covering doctor would likely have thought the same and instructed him to go to the emergency room. There John would have gotten an MRI of his brain, a cocktail of medications to bring his blood pressure down, and another cocktail of medications for his headache. It would be a costly, temporary solution, derailing the long-term one he really needed.

Indeed, I learned that before John was a patient at SCC, he visited the emergency room three to four times every month. During each visit, serious problems were ruled out, but John made no real progress in his overall health. Now, in an incredible turn, he hadn't been to an emergency room since joining the clinic. This was possible because of another key change in the practice model: the doctors at SCC took calls twenty-four hours a day, seven days a week on their own patients.

After-hours calls typically rotate among multiple doctors. They don't know one another's patients. Sometimes they don't even share electronic medical records. This leads to suboptimal behaviors like scrambling to catch up to a medical story and risk aversion when uncertainty exists. One of my patients is a middle-aged woman with a history of breast cancer, an intestinal disease called diverticulitis, and chronic pain that has led to a dependence on opioids. I was out of the office one day when she called, noting pain in her abdomen in the same spot where she had diverticulitis before. The on-call doctor sent her to the emergency room where she received high doses of opioids before a CT scan ultimately showed no diverticulitis. It made sense in the moment for a doctor who didn't know her but set back the slow and steady progress we had made on tapering her pain medications.

I could relate. Many times I have sent my colleagues' patients to the emergency room or was quicker to overtreat the potential worst-case scenarios when I was the one covering. Sending a patient to the emergency room or prescribing antibiotics or pain medications "just in case" always makes sense in the moment when you lack the ability to say, "Tell me how you're feeling tomorrow." The problem is a default that manufactures this moment over and over.

Still, being on call all the time sounded draining. I asked Cuan and Vollrath how they felt about the schedule. They averaged just one to three calls a week, they told me. Cuan extolled the benefits of knowing the callers, telling me about one man with Parkinson's disease whose blood pressure often plummeted while standing. Previously, he had gone to the emergency room three or four times a *week*. "It takes a comfort level of me knowing him and having that experience with him to say, 'Start these medications; let me know if it gets worse.'" Vollrath told me that over her nine years with SCC, she had been awakened only four times. "It was pretty sustainable," she said. "It's not like I had to open Epic." And while she occasionally got calls when hiking with her family on weekends, she assured me she didn't mind: "My kids were at an age when they didn't want to talk to me."

After the occupational therapist finished the Feldenkrais exercises with John, I shadowed other team members. I joined the social worker as she gently and methodically helped a patient connect her binge-eating impulses to childhood trauma. I watched the pharmacist work to eliminate an older patient's dizziness by paring down a mix of pills that had accumulated from multiple doctors. I watched the nutritionist go into more detail about a low-sodium diet for a patient with heart failure than I ever could.

As the day wound down, team members reconvened in the main room. They discussed their shared patients. They tied up loose ends. They even took the time to debrief with me. As I headed home, I felt strangely calm. My day had been so different from the hectic routine I was used to that I felt as if I'd walked into a different job altogether.

MY DAY WITH STANFORD COORDINATED CARE felt great. Here was a clinic that managed to create the nonfragmented relationships with patients I had been seeking for so long. But a practical question loomed: did that translate into better medical care?

From the get-go, Glaseroff and Lindsay knew they needed to test this. The question was how. Proving that primary care "works" is tricky. Surveying patient satisfaction is one option, but everyone knows doctors who are more beloved by patients for their personality than their clinical know-how. The team wanted to find meaningful indicators that the SCC methods were working.

They decided to look at objective markers of health. These included blood and urine test results in patients with diabetes to assess diabetic damage, blood pressure readings in patients with hypertension, and whether patients underwent routine cancer screenings such as mammograms and Pap smears. They worked with Epic to color-code each patient's results into a visual dashboard in their electronic chart. A green result for a particular value meant the patient was at goal, yellow meant room for improvement, and red meant the danger zone.

Experts have a name for tying financial incentives to how *well* patients do based on metrics like these compared to how *much* medical care they receive: value-based care. Sometimes incentives are doled out in traditional fee-for-service practices as annual performance bonuses for physicians. Other clinics eradicate fee-for-service entirely and incorporate value into a broader payment model that holds a health care organization fiscally responsible for patient outcomes. The idea is that clinics should be incentivized and rewarded for coming up with ways to improve patients' health. Tracking metrics is the first step.

The color-coded markers used in SCC didn't just help the doctors understand their patients' gaps; they also turned into motivators for the patients. "I would give it [to patients] without comment and say, 'Here's your data; let me know if you have questions,'" Glaseroff told me. "They'd ask, 'What's this red stuff?' and I'd say, 'It means a high risk of bad stuff happening.' And they'd go, 'How do I get rid of it?'" That exchange was much more effective "than walking into a clinic room and saying 'you're a bad patient,' which is generally what happens," he said.

This approach built off the ideas of Kate Lorig, professor emeritus at Stanford Medicine, who as a graduate student invented a chronic disease self-management program for patients that has since expanded internationally. She described the concept to me over a phone call: "We put people with all kinds of chronic conditions together in the same workshop," she said. The paradigm-changing part of her work was recognizing that most of chronic illness management is done by the patient outside the doctor's office. The medical system had to move past lecturing, she believed, to teaching people to identify challenges and solve problems associated with their illnesses.

This may sound self-evident now. But it was not at all obvious in the year 1978 when she started saying it. And even today, our medical system rarely incorporates this logic. Take, for example, a patient struggling with weight loss. As a doctor, how do you help him? Short of weight-loss surgeries or prescription medications in rare cases, our current system says a doctor should schedule a twenty-minute visit to discuss eating less and exercising more, then rinse and repeat every year.

Does it work? Usually the answer is no. So what does work? First, patients must be in a place in their lives where they feel able, ready, and motivated to make changes. Then the goal is to achieve long-term changes in decreasing food intake and sticking to healthier options, increasing exercise, and avoiding cues that promote habits like excess snacking. Studies have verified that the most effective "treatment" for weight loss is learning these concepts in programs conducted by trained staff (who do not need to be MDs) and by self-help groups.

As Lorig, who shared that she was born with an illness called Gaucher disease, a condition in which her body lacks an enzyme to break down lipids, told me, "Everybody self-manages. You cannot *not* self-manage. It's whether you do it well or you do it poorly."

With this philosophy in mind, Stanford Coordinated Care found that when patients lead the charge, the results can be remarkable: the metrics they collected on exceedingly complex patients somehow became a sea of green. Glaseroff shared one success story with me about a patient with Parkinson's disease who used to love long-distance running. Glaseroff asked him, "Why can't you run?" Apparently, the man looked at the doctor like he was crazy. "Can't you see? I have Parkinson's; my feet hurt even when I walk." A bit of investigation revealed why: as the patient grew older, the arches of his feet relaxed. Because he had continued to wear the same shoe size, his toenails were getting crushed. The clinic encouraged him to buy a larger pair of sneakers. The rest they put to him:

"What's your action plan?" The patient decided he would first jog around the park across from his house. "OK," they said, "we'll call you and see how it went." ("Always follow up action plans," Glaseroff told me. "That means on the order of a week, not 'see you in three months.'") So a care coordinator called the patient the next day. The jog went fine. "What's next?" "I'll go around twice, every other day," the man decided. That went fine, too. A year later, he ran an eight-mile race.

INNOVATIVE PRIMARY CARE CLINICS by definition are not formulaic. Yet there do seem to be patterns that work: minimizing fee-for-service, lump-sum payments upfront, regular check-ins, team-based care, and tracking healthier outcomes. While most primary care clinics fragment relationships into irregular transactions, places like SCC show that it's possible to create a medical world in which doctors know their patients, patients can access their doctors, and teams work together toward improving health. It makes you wonder why models like this aren't spreading.

I asked that question of everyone I spoke to. "They are spreading," Glaseroff answered. In 2013 fee-for-service was the dominant payment model among nearly 95 percent of all physician office visits. In 2016 it reached its lowest at 83.6 percent (and has since crept back up a few percentage points). SCC has hosted many boot camps for other health care teams to visit, learn, and bring the model elsewhere. As of 2021, innovation in primary care captures one of the largest sectors for venture and private equity dollars in health care.

But even if the arc is positive, change has been slow. A practical challenge is getting an upfront investment predicated on a promise: reduced costs and improved outcomes in the long term. "It took a lot of negotiating and organizing," Cuan said of obtaining

SCC's insurance support. Even when those promises are met, clinics that go against the grain still struggle. In 2021 internal considerations on resource allocation led to a restructuring of Stanford Coordinated Care that removed many of its most unique elements. "It's sad to say," Vollrath told me a few months later, "but [SCC] was probably the best experience of my career. I will not be able to replicate anything like that."

Stanford Coordinated Care got off the ground by convincing the insurance company that paying now would be worth it later. Another idea? Get that lump sum not from insurance companies but from patients. Concierge medicine clinics ask patients to pay monthly or annual fees as though they're enrolling in a gym membership. A more radical model, called direct primary care, runs completely off patient fees and doesn't accept insurance at all, allowing the clinics to machete administrative burdens. The extra funding in both models allows primary care doctors to see fewer patients—capping their practices in the hundreds compared to the standard two thousand-plus—and thus be more accessible to communicate with their established patients.

One friend who left standard primary care for concierge medicine tells me about spending one or two hours with each patient, following them in and out of the hospital, and even having time for home visits. Like Cuan and Vollrath, she gladly accepts being on constant call for the benefit of knowing her patients and taking full responsibility for their care. Her patients adore her. The only downside, she freely admits, is feeling conflicted about serving only patients in higher-income brackets. Indeed, it feels like a crude and limited solution, not to mention inequitable, to ask patients to pay a monthly premium to an insurance company to guarantee medical access only to require them to pay an additional monthly fee to ensure that care is up to snuff.

To revamp primary care more broadly, shifting the payment structure away from fee-for-service is a start, but it's not enough.

Health care spending overall has to match the reality of medical contributions. That means that primary care—which does the bulk of keeping people healthy—needs more funding, period. Other industrialized countries invest an average of 14 percent of total health care spending on primary care—double to triple the portion of spending in the United States. The positive spin on these numbers is that even a small reallocation in spending can go a long way.

Finally, we need to support primary care innovation that focuses on different patient populations—whether it be frail older individuals, people with cancer, people on dialysis, people with mental illness or substance use disorders, or what have you. Models like SCC have identified many services for chronically ill patients, including health coaching, social work, and nutrition. Later they incorporated a librarian who pulled articles in real time for patients or staff who wanted to learn more about a health condition. Other clinics are experimenting with services like transportation to clinic visits, acupuncture, and optometry. We can imagine models that incorporate even more: home visits, dental cleanings, hearing aids, addiction counseling. The potential for what falls under the umbrella of primary care is exhilarating.

Of course execution is everything. A business model is just a business model, and innovation and implementation are two very different beasts. When I was brainstorming about my own practice, I came across medical start-ups that looked great on paper, but when I dug deeper reeked of hidden fees, disorganized phone trees, or struggles to recruit and retain physicians. The culture of an organization matters tremendously, and good leadership sets the tone. The doctors at SCC were an example of this. Four years after I shadowed Cuan, she asked me, "Do you remember the jar?" I didn't. Every Friday morning, she reminded me, the team sat around the center table and took turns pulling folded papers from a jar to which they all contributed. On each slip of paper was a compliment.

Thinking about how models that work will spread, I kept returning to a point Glaseroff made. "It's about aligning incentives," he said. "If you have an organization where financial success is based on people not going to the emergency room, the system will come up with an answer." I thought about aligned incentives on multiple levels: between patient and doctor, between doctor and health care organization, and between organization and payer. Just as a doctor saying "stop smoking" to a patient doesn't work, neither does a CEO saying to doctors "work harder." Patients need to help steer their own health, and doctors need to be at the helm to reinvent healthier systems. Too often health care is portrayed as a battle of trade-offs: we want better health, high patient satisfaction, and lower costs, but something has to give. Models like SCC, however, show that truly unified primary care is actually how we win on all fronts.

I think about this a lot in my own practice, where I aim to provide this kind of complete care but run up against a fragmented system every day. I accept that there are some things I cannot change right now. My schedule remains booked with back-to-back patient visits. My Epic InBasket is always overflowing. I take plenty of work home with me. I cannot create physical spaces from scratch, which means that connecting my patients with other providers requires sending them to another building on another day, sometimes months later.

But what I lack in time and shared space, I have gained in continuity. About a year ago, a colleague asked if I could take on a patient of his, a lymphoma survivor, with whom quite frankly he was fed up. I clicked through the patient's records and got a glimpse of why. I gleaned that she doctor-shopped, seeing many doctors a handful of times after which she either dropped them or they dropped her. During our first visit, I considered beginning to address a long list of medical issues. But instead I tried something different. I asked her to tell me about herself. She seemed surprised but went with it. She told me about growing up in a small town where the only doctor around started her on intravenous medications she was later told may not have been necessary. This broke her trust in health care. She shared about the death of her mother and brother the same year and how that made it easy to fall down some dark roads. We used that thirty minutes to plant the seeds of trust I hoped would help us next time in unexpected ways. That was the beautiful thing about being her primary doctor; I knew there *would* be a next time.

Over the past year, I have had the immense privilege of watching her health and well-being blossom. My patient's cancer remains cured, she is on a stable medication regimen, and every visit she brings her journal to show me the many steps she has taken to improve her own health. I appreciate the irony. In a fee-for-service world, what I did during that initial visit would be ranked close to nothing; I prescribed no medications, ordered no tests, and did no procedures. It turns out that doing nothing was the foundation for everything else.

Part 3

The Stories
We Tell
Ourselves

Chapter 7

These Things Happen

FEBRUARY 23, 2016—THE DAY THAT SPLIT MY LIFE INTO before and after—began as a call day on the hospital wards. My pager continued to buzz. Mr. R wanted to talk to the doctor. Could Ms. K have some medicine for her pain? There was a new admission from the emergency room. It was busy, which was normal. I was seven months into my residency, and as busy as it was, I loved it. I loved being a doctor.

Then my mom called. When I picked up, I couldn't make out what she was saying. She was screaming.

"Chest compressions?" I repeated the last phrase I thought I'd deciphered. I paused, in disbelief.

A doctor was on the line next. "Please talk to my daughter; she's a doctor," I heard my mother explain in the background.

The doctor spoke in numbers. My father's sudden cardiac arrest lasted twenty minutes. Nine electric shocks were administered. Six ribs were broken. He was put on two vasopressors and three antibiotics. He had one breathing tube down his throat.

I was afraid these details were a prelude to something I could not bear to hear. I steadied myself on a nurses' station and interrupted with the only question that ever mattered: "Is my dad alive?"

As thankful as I was that the answer to my question was "yes," my father was in critical condition and hardly out of the woods. Next came an avalanche of setbacks, complications, and uncertainties. Suddenly, my sister and I, both physicians, were transported to the other side of the medical interaction: we had become grieving family members. We trod an uncomfortable middle ground, knowing enough to have opinions on our father's medical care and invested enough to advocate for what we felt he needed, but we also felt powerless, pushed to the medical sidelines. For the next two months, our mental energy was spent not only on grieving but also on the politics of questioning our father's doctors.

My father's doctors were blocked from seeing his full story by the same obstacles of fragmentation I knew well: piecemeal medical records, cumbersome electronic charts, and patchy scheduling. But as I sat by my father's side nearly twenty-four hours a day, I saw another narrative. I saw how fragmentation can creep from *within* medical culture: as a mindset that is taught, reinforced, and perpetuated, even subconsciously. I watched a medical team respond to the snapshot of his story that was loudest in the moment—fragmenting decision-making into a series of short-term, reactive choices, abstracted from the past and future of the patient's larger narrative. I witnessed how, locked in this mindset, his medical team dealt with complications when they arose instead of working to prevent them. So the complications snowballed, all while being accepted as par for the course.

My time on the inside had given me clues for navigating some of the hardest choices imaginable with limited information. The question now was whether any of it would make a difference.

I KNEW SOMETHING WAS WRONG when I woke up that morning. I looked at my phone's notifications and saw several missed calls and text messages from my mom. Between how busy she knew my schedule was and the three-hour time difference between California and my parents' home in New York, I knew she wouldn't have called me at 6:00 a.m. my time if it weren't important.

"Something strange is happening with Dad," she started when I called back. It began the evening before. My father's hands were shaking at the dinner table. Then after dinner, while he stayed to clean up and my mom was in another room, he fell from his chair and was too weak to stand back up. He was on our kitchen floor for about an hour before my mom found him. They both thought he needed some sleep. But the next morning, too weak to get to the bathroom, he wet the bed.

None of this was ordinary. My father was sixty-eight years old at the time and relatively healthy. He worked full time as a statistics professor and regularly commuted from home in Long Island through the streets of New York City, heavy briefcases in hand. His classes ran four hours long, and he would stand the whole time save for a fifteen-minute break. Shaking, falling, weakness, and incontinence were all sudden and concerning changes.

I had triaged calls like this from patients many times, but my voice shook as I asked my mom to put my dad on the phone. The range of possibilities ran through my mind, but one thing was clear: my father was sick, and it couldn't wait.

"Dad, I'm sorry to do this to you, but you have to go to the emergency room," I said. My father agreed to do whatever I thought was best. My mom then called an ambulance, as my father was too weak to get in our car.

Then I went to work. I juggled caring for my eight hospitalized patients with answering texts from my mom. I learned that my father was experiencing an irregular heart rhythm called atrial fibrillation. He was spiking fevers. Blood work in the emergency room showed that his potassium level was low and his white blood cells were high. High levels of an enzyme called creatine kinase suggested a muscle injury. "He's getting admitted to the hospital," my mom texted next.

I spoke briefly to the admitting doctor on the phone. My dad had what looked like a urinary tract infection and possible pneumonia. They were getting a head CT scan to rule out a bleed after the fall in our kitchen. He would be in the hospital for a few days. The doctor was curt, and I spoke quickly to interject other salient parts of my father's story and rattle off a few more suggestions. I didn't want to micromanage another doctor's care, but I also needed to advocate for my dad.

A few hours later, just after 2:00 p.m. my time, the call came from my mom—the worst call. My father had just returned from getting the CT scan when a nurse noticed he was still. He wasn't breathing. His pulse was gone. A code blue was called, and a crowd descended to try to resuscitate him while my mother screamed outside the door.

My hospital, too, is loud and chaotic, and I initially caught every other word as I pressed the phone to my ear and ran down the hospital hallway to find a better spot. I ran past nurses I knew and past patient rooms I had just visited, tears running down my face, until I finally leaned on a nurses' station for support.

For a doctor, learning to run a code blue for a sudden cardiac arrest—the ultimate medical emergency—is a rite of passage. When a sudden cardiac arrest occurs outside a health care setting, the chances of survival are an abysmal 10 percent. Within the hospital, that number remains less than 25 percent. Trying to bring a person back to life requires aggressive measures. Health care workers lock their fists and pound on a patient's rib cage with an intensity that often shatters bone (explaining my father's six broken ribs). Electric shocks send an unconscious body careening into the air. A doctor at the head of the bed inserts a breathing tube. Every couple of minutes, a team member feels for a pulse. If it does not return after a certain number of cycles, the team leader must make the ultimate decision of whether to stop everything and pronounce the patient deceased. Imagining the scene with my father at the center felt impossible.

I found a bench outside and absorbed the awful details while nurses ate their lunches several feet away. I knew the next call I had to make. My sister, Shara, was a doctor doing her first year of residency at a hospital in New Jersey about an hour and a half from our parents. She knew that our father was in the emergency room, but now I had to pass on the update.

"Dad's . . . alive," I said, searching for the right words. I hated hearing from my sister what my mother must have heard from me. She collapsed into tears, and I heard her explain to her medical team that she had to go. Then I did the same to my colleagues, who took my pager and offered to cover my patients for as long as I needed. I headed to the airport and bought a ticket for a red-eye to New York. For six long hours on the plane, I drifted in and out of sleep. I was trying to prepare mentally for what might await me when we landed.

When I arrived at the hospital the next morning, I took a deep breath before entering my father's room. My mother and sister were inside, and my sister began giving me updates. She was mid-sentence when she registered what I looked like and stopped. I was looking at my father, and I had begun to cry. My dad looked like my sickest patients: plastic breathing tube taped to his cheeks, chest rising and falling rhythmically with the ventilator, catheters inserted into his arms as bags of medications dripped into his veins. It was an image of life support.

I touched his shoulder. "Dad?" My father opened his eyes. He looked at me, took my hand in one of his, and placed his other hand over his heart. He couldn't speak on the ventilator, but the gesture was clear: he was grateful to see me. I told him I was glad I was there, that we would do everything we could to help him get better, and that I loved him. He continued to hold my hand, nodding.

My father had survived the code. When I felt him squeeze my hand that morning, I thought, "It's bad, but the worst is over." I was wrong.

❖

IT IS A PROFOUNDLY UNCOMFORTABLE and often terrifying experience to be on a ventilator. A tube is down your throat, connecting you to a machine that controls your every breath. You cannot
speak. You cannot inhale or exhale on your own. Some survivors
describe the experience as feeling like suffocating. So it's standard
medical practice to sedate patients who are intubated to relieve
their discomfort. It's also standard to use the minimum sedation
necessary to achieve the desired effect.

For the first two days, my father required minimal sedation
and found other ways to communicate without his voice. He gave
nurses and doctors a thumbs-up. He wrote to us on scraps of paper,
sharing how he felt and asking us to call his university and cancel
his classes. It pained me to see him like this, but I felt cautiously
optimistic that he was able to communicate so clearly so soon after
a cardiac arrest.

My father was critically ill, with a weakened heart, liver damage, and kidney failure from the cardiac arrest. He continued to
spike high fevers, suggesting he was still suffering from an infection. But tests revealed that his lungs were spared from the damage, thus meeting one of two criteria to be successfully taken off a
ventilator. The other criterion is that a patient needs to be awake,
so they can cough and clear the respiratory secretions that natu-
rally build up.

By all accounts, my father was meeting both criteria. During
morning rounds on the third day after his cardiac arrest, his medical team discussed removing his breathing tube. But by that evening, the team had left, and the breathing tube remained. The
evening nurse watched him writhing in discomfort as the sedation
meant to keep him calm wore off. She had a doctor's order in the
form of a range: sedate to keep comfortable. "Can we remove the

breathing tube now?" I asked. "No, the covering doctor is busy," the nurse replied. It would have to wait until tomorrow.

"I don't want him to be uncomfortable tonight," the nurse said, and my sister and I nodded. "But please," I suggested—trying, as I would so many times over those months, not to overstep—"please, minimal sedation. He needs to be awake in the morning."

The next day, my father could not be aroused. He was "semi-comatose," as his team put it, and he stayed that way all day. Our explanation was that his kidneys, significantly weakened from the cardiac arrest, were slow to clear the high-dose sedative drip that had been infused throughout the night.

"We can't pull the breathing tube when he's like this," his doctors said. "He needs to be awake so he can cough and protect his airway."

One day seemed to change everything about how his medical team viewed his story. All the other facts of critical illness after a cardiac arrest persisted. Blood test results indicating a liver injury skyrocketed. His kidneys continued to fail, and he was started on dialysis. He needed two continuous infusions of medications just to keep his blood pressure within a safe range.

Now, on top of all that, my father wasn't waking up. The difference in imagery was striking. Before, when he was a patient writing messages to his family, such a collection of findings could be interpreted as very serious but potentially solvable. But this one additional factor seemed to transform the likelihood of my father's recovery in his medical team's eyes from possible to unrealistic.

As my father's doctors rotated, my family did our best to convey the story to each concerned new face, sharing that my father was awake and communicating with us after the cardiac arrest. When the infectious diseases doctor came in, I asked about broadening the antibiotics. I was worried that the infection that may have provoked the cardiac arrest was not being fully treated. The doctor responded by putting his hand on my shoulder. "I'm worried about him," he said. I was silenced. As a doctor, I knew those words well. They are words I've used countless times. They mean I'm worried a patient will not survive.

The next day, as my father continued to lie motionless, my sister and I strategized before the hospital rounds began. We were afraid of what was coming. What if they recommend stopping treatment and shifting focus toward making him comfortable to die?

The team came in and told us what I had feared: things were bad, and they were very, *very* worried. I'll never know if they were going to take the conversation one step further because I jumped in and made our case. I remember the social worker staring at me, her eyes sympathetic and her brow furrowed. *That poor family,* her expression seemed to say, *in denial about what is happening.* But at that moment, with my doctor mind front and center, I didn't want sympathy. I wanted more time for my dad's kidneys and liver to heal and to clear the sedatives. I wanted broad-spectrum antibiotics. I wanted a CT scan of his chest, abdomen, and pelvis to search for sites of infection we could be missing. I wanted everything I would do for my own patients before declaring that we had tried everything.

Perhaps some doctors thought we were in denial or were displeased with our interjection. But soon one doctor was nodding and then another. Finally, the team leader, the cardiac care unit attending—to whom I'm forever grateful—agreed.

They ran the tests. My father's blood cultures and urine culture came back showing rare bacteria that were often resistant to standard antibiotics, validating our request to broaden his treatment. The CT scan didn't show any sites of additional infection. One of the residents we liked best came to tell us the news. He handed me a folded piece of paper: it was a copy of the radiology report.

"You found this," he said. He was speaking in a low voice, and it struck me even then how strange it was that it was taboo to hand patients and their families their own medical data. This was before the Cures Act Final Rule mandated that patients and their loved ones are privy to their own medical stories. For so long, that was the culture, and I understood.

"Thank you," I whispered.

THE DOCTOR WHO WROTE my father's sedative order as a range had reasonably offloaded one decision to an experienced ICU nurse, and the nurse who sedated my father had good intentions. Given the picture—an uncomfortable patient grimacing on a ventilator—a natural response was to do as she did. But the aftermath of her choice in that one moment was significant, as the sedation took days to wear off, complicated the team's perception of my father's prognosis, and set the stage for other, preventable complications. I began to think back to other instances of health care workers reacting to a fragment of a patient's story in the moment, with damaging downstream effects.

One time I was working in the hospital overnight when a man with a bone marrow disease that had spread to his kidneys was getting worse by the hour. He became more and more somnolent, and soon he was in a deep sleep. Calling his name did nothing. Even rubbing his sternum hard didn't cause him to rouse. The primary resident called the ICU fellow: "He needs to be intubated," the resident explained. His concern was that the patient was too sleepy to cough and protect his airway. But when the ICU fellow came by and reviewed his case, she had a different take. "This is ridiculous," I remember her saying. "He is somnolent because he's in kidney failure. He needs *dialysis*, not intubation." We placed a catheter and started urgent dialysis overnight, and over the next few hours he began to wake up. He was spared an intubation—a serious, risky, and invasive procedure—that could have led to many other problems.

In another situation, I was part of a team caring for a sixty-year-old woman with metastatic breast cancer who was recovering from a major operation to open a blockage in her intestines. In the middle of the night, the doctor was called because of an extremely fast heart rate. He printed out an ECG, determined that this was a heart rhythm called atrial tachycardia, and prescribed a beta-blocker medication to slow it down. For days this pattern continued. Every day the patient's pulse soared, while a doctor focused on the finding that summoned her and gave either IV fluids or beta-blockers to slow it. But days later, a vaguely distended abdomen on the patient's physical exam prompted us to dig deeper: *why* was the patient flipping into this heart rhythm? We wheeled her to the CT scanner and identified the infection in her abdomen that was causing her pulse to soar. We treated an infection, and the heart rate issue resolved.

Finally, I was working on the hospital wards one morning when lab tests showed that the red blood cell count of one of our patients had dropped dramatically. He needs a blood transfusion, my intern suggested, and a colonoscopy to evaluate for a gastrointestinal bleed, which he has suffered before. The intern called the nurse to place two large-bore IVs and called the blood bank to mobilize a transfusion. She called a gastroenterologist and ordered the giant jug of laxative to the patient's bedside for the colonoscopy's preparation. But when we reconvened in the afternoon and ran through our patient list, we looked through the chart and noted that the overnight doctor started our patient on continuous IV fluids to respond to low urine output. Could his red blood cell count have dropped not because he was losing blood but from fluids diluting the number? We quickly changed course, stopping the fluids, waiting, and checking again in twelve hours. Sure enough, his blood counts improved.

What do these stories have in common? Doctors learn that good medicine is responding quickly and decisively to the clinical picture in front of you. Is the patient uncomfortable on a ventilator? The solution: sedate. Is there a fast heart rate? Slow it down. What about a low blood count? Transfuse. But these stories show how even highly trained professionals can be effortlessly led off course by reacting to a momentary picture at the expense of a larger story. I've seen—and been complicit in—knee-jerk reactivity that places patients on a conveyor belt of predictable "fixes" that miss the larger problem. The real answer is for doctors to pause and look for the bigger picture.

Let me be clear: medicine is incredibly difficult. As doctors we make hundreds of decisions a day. Multiple problems present themselves at once, in different states of diagnostic uncertainty. We are bombarded with details that turn out to be red herrings. Sometimes the urgency of a problem is so high that we must act, even while the full story is not yet in focus. There is no doubt that it is partly because doctors face so many decisions that we develop an attitude to touch it once—that is, make a decision and move on. But as medicine rewards reacting quickly and decisively to a fragment of a story—even though it may mean getting it wrong—it raises the question: can taking a step back to view a fuller picture be taught, too?

BACK AT MY FATHER'S BEDSIDE, it was day seven after the cardiac arrest. His fevers were abating. His liver was improving. But one thing remained as terrifying as ever: he still wasn't waking up. Every day my family drove to the hospital and spent the day sitting next to him. Every night we drove home feeling more and more dejected.

Was this still the result of that one night of sedation? As the days passed, it became harder to ignore the worst-case scenario: that lack of oxygen during the cardiac arrest had left him with a brain injury. The medical team consulted the neurology team, who ordered a head CT to look for brain swelling and placed electrodes on his scalp for an electroencephalogram (EEG) that would evaluate the possibility that he was having seizures.

For days my dad was so physically close to me and yet infinitely far. I felt my world divide in two, just as it had during the initial cardiac arrest. What difference did it make that an infection was improving if my dad couldn't wake up?

Around 11:00 p.m., my mom and I sat by my dad's bedside, waiting for the results of the head CT. A resident entered the room. She was new to us.

"The CT scan was normal," she started. I let out a long breath. My mother and I hugged, gratitude moistening our eyes.

"But I'm looking at the patient," the resident continued, "and it's not promising."

My mom started. "What do you mean, 'not promising' "?

I began to ask the doctor questions. How do we interpret the fact that he was communicating right after the cardiac arrest? How do we think about anoxic brain injury with so many confounders, like sepsis, oversedation, and metabolic disturbances from renal failure? What was the result of the EEG?

I wasn't trying to quiz her, but it became apparent that I couldn't trust her. She didn't know that my father was awake for two days after the code. She didn't know about the sedation. She was unfamiliar with his kidney injury. Because she didn't know the full story, she floundered and backtracked about the details but somehow only became more resolute in her conclusion that my father would never wake up.

After she left, I spent a lot of time reassuring my mother that it wasn't true.

I don't envy the position that doctor was in. She had just rotated on, her to-do list was probably a mile long, and first on it was to tell a family she didn't know about the CT results of a patient she was still learning about. And by the way, the daughters are both physicians.

As an individual, she was not responsible for the fragmented external circumstances that placed her in this position. And I can imagine how her choice to speculate beyond the CT scan was shaped by a cultural attitude that I'd been taught, too: the picture of the patient in front of you matters most. But in this case, the effect of anchoring on this one fragment of my father's story—and then choosing to close the door on the entirety of his life—was as hurtful as it was untrue.

I happened to be there alone when my dad's arms started to move. The respiratory therapist came in and checked the ventilator settings. My father was fighting the machine, he noted. I realized that any new team member coming into the middle of this story could look at this picture and believe the right move would be to sedate my father again. So I stayed, fortifying my will to prevent this.

By the next day, he was moving more. "Dad, Dad, Dad, it's me, Ilana, can you hear me?" He moved his head up and down. "Dad, can you wiggle your toes?" He did.

After nearly another full day of this, he finally opened his eyes. We looked at each other. "Dad, we're going to find someone to remove the breathing tube," I assured him.

My mother successfully summoned one of the ICU fellows, who came by later that day and ran standard tests for lung function and alertness. My father passed with flying colors. "Can you cough?" And the tube was out. My dad looked exhausted. He had spent nine days on a ventilator, most of them semicomatose. The fellow began to assess his awareness. My mom sat on one side of the room. The fellow pointed to my sister and me, seated on the other: "Who are they?"

"My daughters," my father said, his voice hoarse and muffled but confident as ever. "Shara and Ilana."

❖

THE REALITY OF MEDICINE is that reacting to one fragment of a patient's story rarely ends there. In addition to the mental toll we endured, the extra days my father spent on the ventilator posed enormous physical risks—respiratory infection, tracheal bleeding, a collapsed lung, or even tracheostomy surgery for long-term breathing support. Though my father narrowly escaped these most serious harms, nine days on the ventilator created very real setbacks. Prolonged insertion of the breathing tube caused his vocal cords to swell, and when it was removed, he had trouble swallowing. He couldn't safely eat or drink without the risk of aspiration into his lungs, so the team inserted a feeding tube through his nostril down to his stomach. The tube provided my father with nutrition, but one of the rotating doctors forgot to order plain water with the feeds to prevent dehydration. The imbalance caused the sodium in my father's bloodstream to shoot up, and he became confused. Every few minutes he asked me for water.

"He is delirious because he is thirsty and hypernatremic," I suggested to his doctors, referring to his high sodium levels. Once I mentioned this, the team did give him some water through the tube. But confusion in a critically ill patient can have a multitude of causes, and the CCU attending had another thought: "Maybe he's confused from uremia," she said, suggesting a buildup of waste products that were not being cleared by his still-healing kidneys. "Let's try dialysis again."

A vascular surgeon came by and inserted a dialysis catheter into my dad's neck. Meanwhile, I was sneaking him ice chips. After a few days, the dialysis wasn't helping, so the doctor on call suggested that the catheter be removed. But it was the weekend, and no one was around to pull it.

"Leaving a catheter in too long can let another infection into his bloodstream," I offered weakly. Though I knew how to remove dialysis catheters, in this hospital I didn't have authorization to do so.

We couldn't let my father develop a catheter-associated infection, I pleaded to myself, because of dialysis, because of confusion, because of high sodium, because of a feeding tube, because of swollen vocal cords, because of nine days on a ventilator, because of oversedation.

Fortunately, no catheter-associated infection developed. But one or two seemingly small missteps quickly turned into problems. Could I attribute all of my dad's complications with 100 percent causality to that night of oversedation? Of course I couldn't. But had it increased his risk of otherwise avoidable complications? Absolutely, yes, it had.

I started to see my father's hospitalization as an endless series of branch points: each of them could make or break the recovery of a critically ill person who was losing the strength to endure an additional setback. His medical care was a game of risk, with many decision points that in the moment could be shrugged off by his medical team as mere details but that could have a profound impact down the line. I felt constantly on the brink, one misstep away from the complication that could sentence him to an unrecoverable doom.

There were near misses that felt only as distant as a blink away. I could imagine the alternative all too clearly because I'd seen it in other patients.

One day, for example, my dad was scheduled to go for a radiology scan that would last for hours. I believed that so soon after a cardiac arrest, he should go with a monitor to check his heart rhythm. But his was missing. For the covering doctor, the short-term calculus was this: my father "had no arrhythmias today," while heart monitors were hard to come by. Send him to the scan and move on.

But I thought back to a story I heard from one of my colleagues: Mr. P, eighty years old and at high risk for arrhythmia, was moved between hospital units without a heart monitor. He lost his pulse on the way. My colleague and her team started chest compressions in the parking lot, but it took several minutes to obtain a monitor from the nearest building and assess his rhythm. He died on the pavement.

At each branch point in my father's case, I struggled to convey to each team member why I was making a big deal out of what seemed like minor, momentary issues. I never imagined that advising my father's medical team would be the role I would step into. I let many things go unmentioned to avoid micromanaging, and I felt uncomfortable every time I noted something I felt was too important to stay silent about. However, as I watched decisions that reacted to a fragment spiral and put my father in harm's way, I had no choice. To become a bystander at this point felt not only irresponsible but impossible.

ULTIMATELY, A BLEED BECAME the final complication that persuaded my family to seek out a different approach. My father had been in the CCU for nearly three weeks. One day, while wearing a hospital gown and sitting in a chair next to his bedside, he moved to stand. We watched as a puddle of bright red blood splattered on the floor. My polite and respectful father was embarrassed, instinctively apologizing to the medical team that rushed in: "I'm sorry, I made a mess."

Every bowel movement thereafter filled the toilet with bright red blood, multiple times a day. His red blood cell count dropped fast, and he needed blood transfusions. The medical team consulted the surgical team, who came to evaluate him.

Their biggest concern was ischemic colitis—including dead

bowel—after the cardiac arrest. Just as my father's liver and kidneys had been injured due to oxygen deprivation during the arrest, they worried that his colon was another casualty. The surgeons discussed a partial colectomy, walking us through what this would entail: an open abdominal surgery, general anesthesia (with another intubation), removal of dead or injured bowel, and reconnection to create a stoma. My father would be left with an ostomy bag dangling from his abdomen to collect stool.

My father's tenuous medical state meant that there was a real, serious risk that he would not survive the operation. The surgery and any additional complications thereafter could also seriously diminish his quality of life down the line.

We were hesitant, and I worried about the consequences of reacting too quickly to the short-term picture of bleeding. It is true that ischemic colitis can lead to dead bowel. In some cases, this can require surgery. But I recalled the patients with ischemic colitis I'd successfully managed with supportive care—that is, providing fluids and blood transfusions as needed—while giving the bowel time to heal on its own. Alternatively, I had sometimes arranged for a colonoscopy first, to see if the bowel was alive, before committing to a surgery to remove it.

Indeed, there is a window of time and certain clues that suggest surgery is best. If you move too soon, you can do something highly risky and unnecessary, with irreversible long-term consequences. But if you wait until it becomes an emergency, you may lose your chance to operate at all—and untreatable dead bowel can become a fatal complication.

As long as my father was stable, we wanted to avoid the operating room. Days passed as I gingerly held my ground against the surgeons who came to check on him. Soon it became a week. When my father continued to bleed, we requested the colonoscopy to help us make the most informed decision we could.

It was then that my family and I talked about another window:

whether he could safely transfer to another hospital. We were—
and always will be—grateful to a team that reacted with the highest levels of expertise to my father's cardiac arrest and saved his life.
But once the emergency had passed and his medical story became
more about the long term, the daily pangs of fighting against reactive, fragmented decisions reminded us that more could still go
wrong. We couldn't afford another oversight that might spiral into
a major setback or worse.

Before his cardiac arrest, my father had been seeing a cardiologist at Columbia. We decided to page him. "Wow," he kept
repeating, as we summarized everything that had transpired with
my father. Then our ask: "Can you accept him for a transfer?"

He could not, he said, as he did not have admitting privileges,
but he would be involved if my father was admitted to Columbia.
"Hope he gets better!" he concluded and hung up.

He had pried the door open a crack. My sister took the next
steps. She wrote down names and phone numbers with clear, simple instructions. She handed them to the doctor covering the CCU
to sign. She wanted to reduce the workload as much as possible for
the overworked doctor, for whom a complicated logistical task in
the midst of a dozen critically ill patients would have been easy and
understandable to decline.

A bed at Columbia opened sooner than we expected. Understandably, my mom was now having second thoughts. She felt the
worst was over and switching to an entirely new hospital was too
risky. There was also the practical matter that Columbia was much
farther from our home on Long Island, meaning her ability to visit
every day would be harder.

The worst *is* over, my sister and I emphasized, but there are still
many decisions yet to make. We have to optimize our chances that
we get them right.

My father was covered in blankets, cold from the blood loss
and the air-conditioned hospital and so many other things he had

endured. But with complete clarity, he looked at my mom and said, "There comes a time when we have to trust them. They know more than we do."

I will always remember those words, the look in his eyes, and the way he reassured my mother. My father had given us the gift of trust. I hoped our instincts were right.

That night my father was strapped into a gurney in an ambulance while my mother, sister, and I crammed in the back around him. The ride was peppered with haunting reminders of normalcy. My father stared out the window and pointed out buildings in New York City. It was painfully easy to imagine an alternative world where the four of us were riding through the city and seeing the sights, but the blaring siren was a loud reality check to our changed lives.

We arrived at Columbia after midnight, and a senior resident came to examine my father. She was outstanding. She had clearly read my father's chart. She turned to me and my sister to fill in certain details. She homed in on the questions of his medical story that remained unresolved. I felt more relaxed immediately.

As the days went by, these feelings intensified. The colonoscopy that was planned earlier was now carefully arranged with layers of backup that recognized the larger story: serious risks associated with the procedure in someone who had recently survived a cardiac arrest. A team of anesthesiologists evaluated my dad before he was sedated, and an operating room was booked. Even seemingly mundane decisions were approached with a much-appreciated foresight. When my father arrived, his feeding tube remained in place, even though by then he could safely swallow on his own. It would have been easy enough to react: "patient passed swallow exam, remove tube." But looking ahead to the four liters of laxatives he would need for the colonoscopy gave his doctors the keener idea to keep the tube in a bit longer. It felt like instead of playing Whac-A-Mole at every finding, his new team more often considered how those findings fit together. This mindset allowed them to identify and avoid potential problems before they arose.

Because of this shift, I was able to go home more and was relieved to step back from medical advising. I felt safe when the day of my father's colonoscopy finally arrived. Even so, when I received a call from an unknown number, a month of being on high alert caused me to grip my phone. It was the gastroenterology fellow. Why was she calling me?

The procedure was over. There was injured tissue, she explained. It looked consistent with ischemic colitis. There were no spots of active bleeding and no dead bowel. I listened for a good sixty seconds before I realized the "but" wasn't coming. I had to learn to recalibrate my reactions to hearing from my father's doctors; just because they were calling me did not mean it was bad news. She was calling because she was a good doctor, and she was keeping us in the loop.

"Will it heal?" I asked.

"It should heal," she said. I pushed the thought of surgery out of my mind.

The details are sharp in a tragedy, but so, too, are they when you turn a corner. A few days later, as his feeding tube was removed and his gut healed, it was as though my father awoke from a long and terrible nightmare. A month of critical illness–induced delirium melted away, allowing the return of the personality we all knew and loved. We sat in his hospital room and talked for hours. I skipped breakfast and lunch, hungrily absorbing his words, laughing for the first time in weeks. At 4:00 p.m. growls emitting from my stomach gave me away. "Go eat something—I'll pay," my dad said.

Over the next week my father's bleeding slowed and then stopped. We discussed with our medical team whether to proceed with a cardiac catheterization to determine whether a blocked vessel caused the initial cardiac arrest. Together we decided the risks outweighed the benefits, and we pursued a gentler stress test to evaluate for blockages instead. He had none. Next he went to the operating room and had a defibrillator placed. This would shock his heart if he ever developed a deadly arrhythmia again.

As we discussed the best ways for him to get stronger, my dad joked—"I go home, and Mom will carry me around the house"— but he was motivated. Nurses cheered as he pulled himself to a stand and walked laps around the hospital wards. He was accepted into an acute rehab facility. My mother took the train to visit him every day, and I booked a flight back to California. For three weeks, my father did physical therapy where he practiced taking the stairs, occupational therapy where he relearned fine motor skills, and speech therapy to strengthen his swallowing. On April 8, forty-five days after he arrived in the emergency room, my father went home.

DURING THE LONG DAYS in my father's hospital room, in the midst of yet another one of his complications, I thought back to a lecture I had heard in medical school. Mark Zeidel, chair of medicine at Beth Israel Deaconess Medical Center, played a clip for us from the 1963 film *It's a Mad, Mad, Mad, Mad World*. In the scene, Ethel Merman's character berates a driver, who flippantly responds after a car accident has taken place that "these things happen." "What kind of an attitude is that, 'These things happen'"? her character rails. "They only happen because this whole country is just full of people who . . . say 'these things happen!'" Tying the lesson to our own field, Zeidel explained that his hospital had dramatically reduced its rates of central line infections by viewing them as preventable and by creating—as the film suggests—a culture of zero tolerance. The hospital simply refused to let them happen.

My father's illness showed me a pervasive, often subconscious attitude toward complications in critically ill patients: that "these things happen." It also showed me that we must reframe that approach.

Changing a medical culture that reacts to a short-term fragment of the patient's story—and then accepts the consequences—to one that thinks ahead, looks for the larger narrative, and views complications as preventable will be hard. Many improvements in the system would have undoubtedly helped my father's team see his big picture more clearly. His doctors could have benefited from electronic charts, for example, that prompted an order for plain water with his tube feeds instead of relying on a doctor to remember and manually enter it separately each time. They would have been helped by an organized medical records system that more clearly displayed how long a patient had been intubated and cumulative doses of medications like sedatives, making it easier to pick up troubling trends. They would have been aided by a schedule that did not include twenty-eight-hour shifts, which translated into different primary doctors daily, motivated not to rock the boat instead of planning a longer-term approach.

However, all of that being true, I believe that looking for the larger story as an individual in this system remains not only possible but teachable. I believe we can foster a culture that encourages doctors to zoom out to see the big picture rather than paper over problems with short-term fixes. We can promote a mindset that looks beyond the moment. Knowing that it's not feasible to get every detail right, how can we more often take into account a broader outlook? How can we cultivate an intentionality to see the full story rather than a reactivity to address the loudest piece of it?

The first change involves recognizing that quick fixes are often not as pressing—nor as immutable—as they may seem. All doctors have participated in situations that trigger running scrubs and pounding clogs like my father's cardiac arrest, and it's crucial to be able to respond appropriately. But outside of these scenarios, it's actually quite rare that doctors must decide in an instant. Doctors who see the full story take the time to do it. And when they don't have all the information they need at their fingertips, they pause, determine what needs to be done now and what can wait, and act accordingly. The doctors I admire most take it upon themselves to find out more, which requires taking the initiative to check back frequently. When a doctor orders a sedative drip, for example, she has a choice: she can let it run until rounds the next morning, or she can check back every few hours, assess the patient, and adjust the drip as needed. When a doctor notes high sodium levels and confusion in a patient, a choice exists here, too: she can chase all possible sources of confusion at once, or she can correct the sodium, check back on the patient's mental status, and adapt. Medical culture can do better to praise close, proactive follow-up. We can promote the courage to change course as the story unfolds instead of champion a decisiveness that is premature and doubles down on missteps.

At the same time, the way doctors speak about patients entrenches norms that influence how we frame our goals and our agency in achieving them. I had cared for enough patients like my father to imagine how we would discuss him: "sixty-eight-year-old male, post cardiac arrest, with course complicated by prolonged ventilation, dysphagia, altered mental status, hypernatremia, and renal failure." His complications would likely be listed just like that: à la carte, in random order, removing any indication of causality in their unfolding. But watching them from the vantage point of his bedside, I was able to see a list of complications as not random, not inevitable, but as outcomes that cascaded from choices.

Whenever doctors use the passive voice to speak of complications—"patient's course was complicated by a prolonged stay on the ventilator"—we subtly enforce norms that accept complications as unfortunate but inescapable. Whenever we describe mishaps in a fragmented laundry list without any indication of cause and effect, we minimize our control to prevent such outcomes.

Overall, it is beneficial that we have moved from a punitive environment that shames providers for everything that goes wrong in a patient's care to one that focuses on systemic barriers. The cultural shift I hope to see among doctors is not about blame but about reclaiming agency for the good of the patient. It's about doctors asking ourselves, every day and with every patient, "What else can we do to optimize this person's trajectory?"

Finally, as we nurture a culture among doctors to look for the larger story, it is imperative to include patients and family members who invariably know details the medical team cannot. Medical culture must eschew the egos within who treat those who offer information or ask questions as "difficult." My family and I got a taste of this harmful attitude when some doctors dismissed our concerns, even as those concerns were being voiced by companion physicians. The doctors in his care who sought out collaboration with us were not simply kinder but were privy to information that helped them make wiser decisions. So what can patients and loved ones do? I am proud of how my family filled the role of keeper of my father's full story: repeating key facts to different team members, gently reminding them to look ahead, and even coordinating communication. Completely aside from the medical insights we had as physicians, this role was invaluable, as we recounted a past we knew better than anyone and advocated for a future we cared about more than anyone.

"These things happen." Instead of submitting to this attitude, what if we—doctors and patients alike—changed one word? What if we declared instead—not with censure or burden but with empowerment—that these things *matter*?

NEAR THE END OF my father's illness, I was eager to apply these lessons to care for patients again. But as I transitioned back to my accustomed side of the stethoscope, I bumped into challenges. Over those initial few days and weeks back in my hospital, I experienced a newfound insecurity as I found myself hesitating amid the usual torrent of decisions. I felt the weight of getting each right, as I grasped in a way that I hadn't fully appreciated before the significance of even those choices that seemed minor. As a doctor, would I prioritize the patient with a high sodium level over the one who was having acute chest pain? Of course not. But as I faced each decision, I imagined how it could go wrong and become the straw that would make or break a patient like my father.

Being back in the very place that reminded me of fresh personal pain was also affecting me deeply. I became something of a compassion automaton, able to extract the most generous lessons from my experiences with my father and give them to my patients. Then I would go home and let sadness swallow me. With my patients' ups and downs, I circled a confusing arc of emotions at work: this is the last place I want to be; this is *exactly* where I want to be.

I knew this had to change. There had to be a way to appreciate the weight of my decisions without being paralyzed by them. There had to be a way to consider a patient's broader story without drowning in indecision.

There was. In hindsight two things helped me find my compass. The first was a text message. On returning to California, I met up with each person who had helped my family. One was a nephrologist who had talked through my father's failing kidneys with me, providing sound advice from across the country. But when I texted him and asked if he could please let me give him a small gift, he said no. His response was something I reread for a long time afterward. "Just find peace with all that happened. And get back on track. Many patients need your help for many years to come. That will be the gift."

The second was reclaiming my haunts. One day, during a few minutes of downtime at the hospital, I deliberately walked down the hallway where I had received the worst phone call of my life. I ended on the bench where I had digested the worst news. I pulled out my phone and called my dad. We chatted for a few minutes. "I don't say it enough," he said—which wasn't true—"but I am so proud of you."

When a doctor is confronted with the trauma of serious illness, I believe it can go in two ways. The sting of memory can push you away from diving too deep into the story of another's sorrow. You may never again want to scrutinize the same test results that portended whether your loved one would survive or try to find the language to convey the depths of uncertainty you have grappled with firsthand. You can compartmentalize your life and your work or even leave your line of work altogether. I understand this and don't judge anyone who makes this choice.

The other option is leaning into it. I wondered if I could blur the lines between the personal and the professional in a healthy way, blending all my experiences into something deeper, more meaningful, and purer. I could submit to our shared fragility with humility. I could find my mission in the challenge to look beyond the moment as much as I could toward seeing, and treating with respect and reverence, every patient's whole being.

Nearly seven years ago, I made a commitment to myself. Maintaining an intentionality to see the patient's long-term narrative, without succumbing to indecision or self-doubt, is one of the hardest things I've had to do as a doctor. I don't trivialize the mental effort required, and I don't pretend any doctor can uphold this mindset at all times. I assert fully that the system must catch up in parallel. And I harbor no illusions that any doctor will get every decision right in the moment; I've been wrong enough to know. My humble request is that doctors strive to consider the complete story over momentary fixes and listen to the patients who remind us to do this—because that is what all patients deserve.

As I sat on the bench that day in 2016 speaking with my father, it didn't take long before my pager went off. A patient and her husband wanted to see me. The results of her biopsy had come back, and they wanted to know what they meant and what to do next. "Dad, I'm sorry, I have to go," I said. I stood up, shoulders back, stethoscope around my neck, not the same, never the same—but ready. I couldn't go backward. I would take everything I had and pay it forward.

Chapter 8

The Likeliest Unlikely

M ANY DOCTORS WORKED ON MY FATHER'S CASE. THE nephrologist paid close attention to his kidney injury and decided when to start and stop dialysis. The surgeon advised about the possible colectomy. The infectious diseases physician analyzed the source of his fevers and managed his antibiotics. Each ICU doctor on call reacted to any complications—an irregular heart rhythm, a plummeting blood pressure—that arose during her or his shift.

None of this is unusual. If you get admitted to any hospital or develop any chronic illness, you'll notice more than one doctor on your team. You might even see a dizzying array of faces like Jin Wong did. As medicine has advanced, doctors have carved out narrower and narrower niches of specialization. According to the Association of Medical Colleges, which oversees much of medical accreditation, physicians can receive board certification to practice in more than 135 specialties and subspecialties. Today there is no way around it: caring for sick patients involves working in teams.

So doctors navigate a sea of interpersonal questions, not only with patients and family members but with one another: How much should you communicate with each member of the health care team? Should you defer to the expertise others bring or try to synthesize differing perspectives? What happens if you disagree?

It's challenging enough to identify and counteract your own

biases as an individual. My father's case exposed the fragmented mindset that reacts to momentary snapshots at the expense of the long-term picture. This is an outlook to which any individual doctor may subconsciously succumb—and any individual doctor can try to overcome.

But as we work together, we may also succumb to fragmentation in teams. As each specialist takes responsibility for one thread of the patient's overall story, theoretically someone should be reconciling these viewpoints and putting it all together. But the nature of teamwork in medicine can diffuse this responsibility. The whole can fall apart, even while each doctor perfectly manages their slice.

Shortly after I returned from my father's bedside, my colleagues and I were put to the test by the case of a woman I'll call Elle Park. Three teams of doctors were on her case. We had identical data and medical records. We shared the same resources at the same hospital. The only difference was the story we told ourselves.

WHEN I MET ELLE, she was doing jumping jacks in her hospital room. She was trying to "stay healthy," she told me, as she knew a long and grueling path awaited her. Two years earlier, when she was fifty-four, months of fatigue prompted a hematologist to conduct a bone marrow biopsy that revealed a slow-growing cancer. Elle opted to hold off on treatment at the time. She felt mostly fine until an assault of fevers and drenching night sweats revealed that her slow-growing cancer had morphed into an aggressive leukemia. Curing it at this stage would require equally aggressive treatment, she was told, and she was now in the hospital to receive that treatment.

From the day I rotated on as her primary physician in the hospital, Elle and I bonded. I learned that she had married her high school sweetheart, and they had identical twin girls who had recently turned twenty. The family lived in a ranch house by a beach a few hours away. "You have to go there sometime," Elle instructed me. She showed me videos on her phone of her surfing with confidence and skill. I told her about the one time I tried and belly-flopped into the ocean.

Elle enjoyed talking about traveling. "Like Gatsby!" she exclaimed, when I told her I was originally from Long Island, though I admitted ignorance about the East Egg and the West Egg. "I want to take the girls to New York for Christmas."

It was August, and we were both quiet for a moment contemplating that prospect. December, in the land of cancer, was a long time away.

But she had enough people focusing on the worst-case scenario. I went with it.

"You know that big tree? The Rockefeller one? You ice skate around it." Her kids would love that, Elle said. They would probably fall down but laugh the whole time.

Elle's talk about travel waned as she experienced the typical setbacks of chemotherapy for acute leukemia. Her blood counts plummeted as the chemotherapy attacked normal bone marrow alongside her cancer, and she became dependent on daily blood transfusions. Her hair thinned and fell out in clumps. One day she broke out in a full-body rash that made her look like she had been bitten by a hundred mosquitoes.

The chemotherapy also severely suppressed her immune system. Her white blood cells, which fight infection, were wiped to nearly zero, and she spiked a fever. We ordered a chest CT scan to rule out pneumonia, but her lungs were fortunately clear. The source of the fever turned out to be a kidney infection that started from a urinary tract infection. We prescribed a heavy course of IV antibiotics to eradicate any lingering bacteria.

Soon after, we did a bone marrow biopsy to see whether the chemotherapy had worked on her leukemia. While there was some improvement, residual cancerous cells remained. The plan for Elle was to stay in the hospital and go straight to a second round of chemotherapy. She was disappointed but braced herself for more.

Again, her white blood cells dropped just as they had started to recover. She spiked another fever. This time a fungal infection called Candida was coursing through her bloodstream. We added antifungal medications to her antibiotics, and the combination made her vomit. Candida can invade the retinas, so we called an ophthalmologist to examine her eyes. We also removed the catheter in her arm as it posed an ongoing risk of seeding her blood with infection.

For about a week, she was doing better. Her blood cultures showed that she was clearing the fungal infection. Her eyes were spared. Her energy improved to the point that she was once again able to get out of bed and do jumping jacks. We chatted about New York and Christmas and the future.

But soon the fevers returned. Elle began to cough, and I ordered another chest CT. When the radiologist calls you directly, it's never good. "Concerning for evolution of a fungal process or possible drug reaction," the radiologist said. "Or this could be DAH." The last possibility filled me with dread. DAH, which stands for diffuse alveolar hemorrhage, is a serious bleed in the small airways of the lungs, and Elle's low platelet count put her at risk. The treatment, however, is steroids, a medication that would further weaken her immune system when she was already immunosuppressed. Steroids would be risky until infection had been either ruled out or fully treated.

I called the infectious diseases team, who recommended we broaden Elle's antifungals to a powerful IV medication called amphotericin, which can be so toxic (we nickname it "amphoterrible") that we run it with fluids before and after to protect the kidneys. We aggressively replenished her electrolytes. Then one afternoon Elle coughed up blood. She opened a tissue to show me the dark purple clumps. I paged the pulmonary doctors to perform a bronchoscopy and lavage, or wash, of her airways to help us diagnose what was going on.

The following day, she was wheeled to the bronchoscopy suite and sedated while the pulmonologist threaded a thin tube with a camera down her throat and into her airways. The images on the screen didn't show obvious anatomical defects, and there were no signs of hemorrhage. Samples were sent off to the lab to be tested for infection.

A few days later, the tests came back negative for multiple bacterial, viral, and fungal infections. I spoke to the infectious diseases team, who emphasized that we were treating Elle with medications that would cover most infections in immunocompromised patients. A lung biopsy might be worthwhile to clarify the diagnosis, they offered. I talked to her outpatient hematologist, who cautioned against giving white cell booster shots to speed her immune recovery, as those could also stimulate leukemia cells. He also noted that the chemotherapy Elle received wouldn't harm the lungs like this. Finally, I called the pulmonary team. Doing another lavage wouldn't help, the on-call doctor said. A biopsy would be better, but with Elle's platelets so low, getting it could cause a bleed. With nothing more to add, the pulmonary team signed off the case.

We were at an impasse. Over the next few days, I cranked up the oxygen delivered through two plastic prongs into Elle's nostrils: two liters, three liters, five liters. One morning I found her leaning forward, elbows bent against her tray table. I called in the nurse, and we swapped out her nasal prongs for a full face mask. "I can't breathe," she wheezed, as we strapped it over her nose and mouth.

For days we stayed the course, even as Elle was undoubtedly getting worse. We deferred to one another's expertise as her health deteriorated.

❖

WHAT WOULD YOU WANT IF time were short? This is a question I have asked hundreds of patients. Conversations about patient wishes in the event of critical illness have become normalized in the last few years, thanks to grassroots efforts and messaging from the medical community and patient advocacy groups. Terms like "advance directive" are part of the general public's vocabulary, and over one-third of the U.S. population has one.

As such, whenever any patient comes into the hospital, the admitting doctor routinely asks the patient her wishes if she were to become much sicker. This discussion is called a "goals of care" conversation and should be documented in the chart for the entire health care team to respect. For the patient, this dialogue usually amounts to answering the following: If your heart stopped, would you want chest compressions and electric shocks to bring you back? If your lungs stopped, would you want to be sedated and placed on a ventilator to breathe? Who would you want to make medical decisions for you if you cannot do it yourself?

I applaud the goals, but short of that last question—which I believe is the most important one—these options can come across as a baffling laundry list, their meaning obscured until someone actually faces the nuances of a dire situation. Prognosis is not set in stone. The medical story evolves. Discussing goals of care in a meaningful way requires readdressing what a person would want when the specifics become clearer.

The time had come to do that for Elle. I looked at her chart and saw that the admitting doctor had documented "full code," meaning Elle wanted us to do everything possible to maintain her life. But now, as a real possibility of respiratory failure and the need for a ventilator loomed, we had to have a full discussion about what that meant.

I gowned, gloved, and knocked on Elle's door. "Come in!" she called out. Elle was lying in bed: thin, pale, and breathing heavily. It was painful to reconcile the picture before me with the memory of the woman doing jumping jacks just a few weeks earlier.

"Can I sit down?" I asked.

"Uh-oh," she said.

I told Elle I wanted to talk about where we were. I said I would be remiss if we didn't talk about what could happen next. I explained that her oxygen levels were worsening, and if the trend continued, the next step would be intubation. I reviewed exactly what that involved—that she would be sedated and unable to speak in the ICU. She'd had no idea.

"I still want to do everything," she said, her breath quickening.

"I understand."

"I'm not ready to die from this."

"I hear you."

Elle looked down, the wig she had begun to wear slipping and revealing stringy wisps of hair underneath. "But we're not there, are we?" She looked at the pictures of her daughters on her bedside table, then locked eyes with me. "Dr. Yurkiewicz—should I be worried?"

I wasn't sure how to answer that.

The truth was I was very worried. I feared that while we continued to lack a clear understanding of the cause of Elle's decline, if she were placed on a ventilator, she would never get off. I could see how it would play out. Her lungs would continue to fail, until eventually her family would be forced to make the excruciating decision of whether to withdraw care. Ultimately, they would realize (or we would convince them) there was no other choice. The breathing tube would come out, and her family would gather around her bedside as she took her final breaths.

Outside Elle's room, I asked for a meeting with the different teams. This was not easy to arrange as every doctor had a different schedule and workflow. But the following afternoon, representatives from each specialty managed to convene along with Elle's bedside nurse. "If we stay the course," I remember saying, "she will go on a ventilator and never come off."

We talked through the details of Elle's case but didn't land on any additional suggestions. She was very sick. We were doing everything we could. There was nothing left to do but wait and see.

PART OF GETTING IT RIGHT IN MEDICINE is knowing when to call for help—and who can help with what. Behind the scenes, I spend about as much time calling other doctors, doing rounds with other doctors, and directly intervening in emergencies with other doctors as I do having face-to-face discussions with patients. We come together, sometimes with colleagues we know well and sometimes with people we've never met, during extraordinarily high-stakes situations. This can foster a kind of closeness that even our loved ones don't understand. It can also set us up for communication errors that chip away at a good outcome. Mastering your own piece of the patient's puzzle is hard enough. Keeping tabs on everyone else adds layers of complexity that can open space for gaps.

Doctors spend many years training to reach their peak of expertise. For me it was fourteen: four years of college, four years of medical school, three years of residency in internal medicine, and three years of fellowship in oncology and hematology. Subspecialties within specialties allow doctors to dive deeper into narrower slices of medicine. At the end of my fourteen years, I had the option—and was highly encouraged—to consider yet another fellowship, one-year long, in bone marrow transplants. Similarly, after spending fourteen years becoming a cardiologist, doctors can pursue fellowships in electrophysiology or interventional cardiology; a fourteen year–trained gastroenterologist can tack on another year to subspecialize in inflammatory bowel disease or endoscopies. A 2019 *New Yorker* cartoon got it right: "Hmm, so the foot guy sent you here. I'm strictly a knee-and-upper-shin guy—you're going to have to see a lower-shin-upper-ankle guy."

This kind of specialization is favored in large swaths of medical culture. The deeper you specialize, the more you're viewed as an expert—and who doesn't want to be an expert? The specialist path also tends to reap greater financial rewards (no small matter when the average debt accumulated from medical school is a little over $200,000, while residents and fellows earn close to a minimum wage). When my fourteen years finally wound to a close, a speaker at my fellowship graduation read a quote suggesting that lack of specialization is the death of an academic career. It was about ten minutes before they announced the next steps each of us was planning in our careers. I knew mine would say I was opening a primary care clinic for cancer survivors—an important role but, gasp, a generalist.

We need specialists. I have a few on hand to whom I regularly turn to answer questions about my patients, and I am always grateful for their input. But something has happened as doctors learn more and more about less and less. Medical specialization doesn't just inform the recommendations we can confidently offer or the procedures we can deftly perform. They influence larger questions of how we view a patient's story. The problem arises when these stories need to come together.

I know this problem intimately because I've played both roles. When I completed my internal medicine residency and a week later became an oncology and hematology fellow, I crossed an invisible line in the hospital—from generalist to specialist. Suddenly, I went from being the one managing the patient's overall care to the one fielding calls and saying, "Thank you for reaching out, but no, this isn't an oncologic or hematologic problem." No matter how fascinating the case was or how much I wanted to help, my first job was to be the gatekeeper for my niche. Sometimes that meant turning cases down or signing off, as the pulmonary team did after Elle's bronchoscopy. Most strikingly, specialization made it easy not to evaluate the whole picture anymore. My first pass over a patient case involved looking for clues that would suggest blood or tumor problems. If I let myself, I could gloss over the rest. I learned that triaging as a specialist didn't entail asking how sick the person was. Rather, the question became, is this something *I* can help with?

The result can be a strange ecosystem in which many individual physicians are thinking logically and even thinking ahead, but no whole ever takes shape. Imagine this scenario, one I've watched unfold many times: A patient's diagnosis isn't clear. The generalist physician calls all the specialists who might be able to help. Each conducts an evaluation and orders some additional tests. Is this neurologic? Probably not, concludes the neurologist. Rheumatologic? Doubtful, says the rheumatologist. Surgical? Not it, says the surgeon.

Each analysis by itself is sound. And playing gatekeeper is an important job. Saying no to antibiotics when there's no evidence of a bacterial infection or deciding that surgery is more likely to cause harm than good are vital and correct roles for a doctor, both for individual patients and from the standpoint of public health.

But taken together, where does that leave us? The answer is, with a patient with no diagnosis, a patient in pain, or a patient deteriorating.

One story that haunts me occurred while I was caring for an older man who came to the hospital with a flare-up of an autoimmune condition that resulted in multiorgan failure. As happened with Elle, his lungs eventually became his most pressing problem. After two weeks on a ventilator, he underwent a tracheostomy for long-term breathing support. But his oxygen needs were rising as serial CT scans showed stubborn white patches in his lungs. We ordered a battery of tests to understand what was causing this, including one for an infection called cytomegalovirus (CMV) that came back positive. I called the infectious diseases doctor and asked his opinion. He told me it was very unlikely that CMV was responsible for the patient's respiratory failure and the treatment for it can hurt the kidneys. "Is that a chance you want to take?" he asked. I listened. I nodded. Less than a week later, the patient coded and died. His family asked for an autopsy. It showed widely disseminated CMV.

The case was presented to our department in a conference that was a safe space for doctors to unpack and learn from poor outcomes. I listened closely as a panel of experts weighed in and offered different opinions on how they would have approached the case. I didn't mention that what haunted me as much as the devastating ending were the words of a hematologist on the case. Her job was to manage the patient's low platelet count. But the CMV diagnosis had caught her eye. What are you going to do about it? she had asked me. She shared a frightening case she had seen years ago of a similar patient who ultimately died. I listened. I nodded. I shared what the infectious diseases specialist had told me, and I deferred to him.

This was a complicated case. Tying the respiratory failure to CMV was an extraordinarily tough call even in retrospect. From the vantage point of the infectious diseases doctor, it was absolutely true that CMV was unlikely the culprit. But only later did I realize the cognitive blind spot in play: what *was* going on? The patient's lungs were failing, and we had no explanation. Only someone looking at the whole story could meaningfully assess the likelihood of CMV because that assessment had to take into account the likelihood of everything else. Whose job was it to do that? I thought about it. Could the hematologist have spoken directly to the infectious diseases doctor? Sure—but I was the primary doctor, and I was responsible for compiling different inputs into a sensible whole. I had failed to take the initiative to bring that gap to the forefront.

It was early in my career, and I learned a powerful lesson. As a doctor, I worked hard to get better by recognizing and correcting the gaps in my own thinking. But now, I realized, this was a gap that only arose in teams, and with teams responsible for so much care, it was as prevalent as it was unintentional. I saw how easily we can get it wrong when each doctor examines a story through her lens of expertise—taking a piece of the whole and looking at one fragment. From each standpoint, a diagnosis may be considered unlikely or a treatment improbable to work. But what if the patient is getting worse? Almost by definition something unlikely is happening. And team or no team, it doesn't mean an individual doctor can't do something about it.

IN ELLE'S CASE, each team of doctors was technically correct. From an infectious diseases perspective, we were already treating the majority of possible infections. From a pulmonary standpoint, another bronchoscopy was unnecessary and a biopsy dangerous. From a hematologic perch, there was no safe way to speed up recovery of Elle's immune function. But three reasonable narratives added up to an unreasonable conclusion. Staying the course was also a choice—and it was clearly the wrong one.

After our team decided to watch and wait, I went home that night and couldn't sleep. I searched the medical journals for reports of lung toxicity from any of the medications Elle received. I found a handful of case reports on pneumonitis from her first chemotherapy round, some so obscure they were decades old. I also read about rare infections of the lungs in immunocompromised patients, and I wondered whether Elle could have picked up any of these. With my internet browser tabs piling up, I made a list of possibilities and combinations of possibilities no matter how remote. I then listed treatment options for Elle that we hadn't already tried.

The next morning, I walked to the radiology reading room and found a different radiologist from the one who had called me with the CT results. "Can we go over a case?" I asked. I summarized Elle's story as the radiologist scrolled through the most recent and an older CT side by side. Light gray patches overtook the black air-spaces of both lungs, showing frighteningly little healthy lung left.

"The report was worsening fungal infection, drug reaction, or DAH," I said. "Can pneumonitis from chemotherapy look like this?"

"Ground-glass opacities are nonspecific," he said slowly, describing the hazy pattern in Elle's lungs. He couldn't say. But based on appearance alone, we couldn't rule pneumonitis out.

Next I texted an infectious diseases doctor I trusted: "Hey, can I run something by you?" I told her Elle's story over the phone, ending with, "I'm not even convinced that it's an infection. But is there any infection we *are* missing?"

She started naming some immediately. The antifungal Elle was on, amphotericin, covered the Candida she already had and many other fungal infections we can see in immunocompromised patients. But certain rarer species would be resistant, she said. She listed their names as I wrote them on a scrap of paper. "What would you need for that? An azole?" I asked, referring to a different class of medications. "Yeah." And then she spoke the words I was used to: "But it's very unlikely."

Two doctors—three counting me—had looked at the same set of facts and come up with different diagnoses. Maybe it was pneumonitis; maybe it was fungus. This may seem surprising. People understandably expect some degree of uniformity in medicine because it is technical and requires extensive training. I have found that some of my patients are discomfited to find that if you poll five doctors, you may get five different opinions.

Experts offer two theories for how doctors can look at the same case and reach different conclusions. One explanation is bias. As a medical student, I took a course on cognitive biases in medicine and learned to recognize common offenders. There's availability bias (coming up with a diagnosis based on a case you've recently seen), confirmation bias (placing undue emphasis on findings that support your hunch), and anchoring (clinging to a diagnosis even in the face of new information).

"Availability bias" was coined by psychologists Daniel Kahneman and Amos Tversky. Kahneman, who won the Nobel Memorial Prize in Economic Sciences, coauthored a book in 2021 with Olivier Sibony and Cass R. Sunstein that posited a second theory for why experts, including doctors, disagree: noise. Whereas bias involves systematically erring in a certain direction, noise occurs when judgments are scattered seemingly at random. In Elle's case, for instance, bias would be at work if her doctors consistently underestimated the role of rare fungal infections and undertreated them. Noise would mean that every case of pneumonia provoked discordant, inconsistent opinions on the likelihood of rare fungal infections. Noise happens because despite all the technical training doctors receive, medicine also involves making individual judgments according to some amorphous combination of knowledge, experience, and intuition. It's a world in which even small perturbations—a recent case we can't get out of our mind, how swamped we are that day, or even whether it's before or after lunch—can shift that judgment.

How do we reduce noise? The authors mention training and assistance from artificial intelligence—and, they say, "the aggregation of multiple expert judgments." In other words, we need second opinions. Adding more judgments to the mix increases the likelihood the truth will come out.

The day Elle told me she wanted to live, even if that meant being on a ventilator, I alerted the on-call ICU fellow that she might need one. When I signed out, I left instructions to the overnight resident to check on her breathing throughout the night. Elle was scared. I was scared. I worried we were running out of time.

❖

THE THEORY OF NOISE postulates that if I called a different infectious diseases doctor or a different pulmonologist, I might get a different opinion on the likelihood of a resistant invasive fungal infection or a lung biopsy's safety. Noise also suggests that getting more opinions would likely help us make a better decision. But it offers little insight into how to resolve these opinions—or *who* should resolve them.

A few years ago, at the suggestion of a friend who didn't work in health care, I picked up *Crucial Conversations*, a best-selling book on communicating effectively when the stakes are high. The authors write that any "set of facts can be used to tell an infinite number of stories." When faced with conflicting narratives, our default response can be silence or violence. Silence is simply letting disagreement persist. Violence is fighting blindly for your opinion without recognizing alternative views. Medicine is a prime substrate for both suboptimal reactions. But there is a third option, the authors write. Those who are best at dialogue assume rational behavior in others. They find a way to slow down and chart an alternative path.

In medicine it looks like this. Imagine the first pass is the generalist calling all the specialists who might be able to help, where every specialist says some version of "but it's unlikely." Often that's that. But in the best-case scenarios, someone pushes. With all the options laid out and none of them good, someone makes it her job to look beyond the narratives for the truth.

Long after I cared for Elle Park, I was on call as a fellow taking hematology consults. One day I was paged about a man in his fifties with a complex medical history that included a precursor to multiple myeloma, a cancer of the plasma cells in the bone marrow. He was now in the hospital with fatigue, unrelenting nausea, and vomiting. He had lost fifty pounds in just a few months.

I looked through the chart and saw that a hematologist-oncologist had already given an appraisal. I read my predecessor's note; in the doctor's evaluation, the patient's symptoms weren't related to his bone marrow disorder. In many cases, that would have been the end of it. But the doctor who paged me wasn't like other doctors. "I know what he said, but this just *feels* like a heme problem," she said. "Can you please take another look?"

Ironically, the way she framed her question was everything doctors are taught not to do. We learn that a good question to a specialist is a specific one. Can you do a bronchoscopy? Do you recommend starting steroids? But her question was a lifeline: I don't know what's going on, but can you help? She didn't have a specific question. What she had was a sick patient and a hunch.

I looked at the patient's blood counts reported in the electronic chart: normal. Then I pulled his blood smear and looked at it under the microscope. At first glance, everything looked fine. I moved to a different section of the slide. Were those abnormal plasma cells? They weren't mentioned in the automatic result reported by the lab. I called another hematologist who had special expertise in plasma cell disorders to look at the case with me. The patient had plasma cell leukemia. It was an extremely rare transformation from his initial disorder that could explain his symptoms; it was missed by the automated blood counts from the computer; and it needed to be treated right away.

The internist who called me succeeded where others can fall short in two ways. First, she refused to accept the narrative when it didn't add up. That insight came from within. Second, she had the communication skills to convince someone else. This is hardly an argument for overstepping or disrespecting expertise. She didn't pretend she knew what a hematologist did about a hematological problem. But she went with her instincts, and her instincts were right. Because of a crucial conversation, the patient's life was saved.

❖

THE MORNING AFTER I TOLD ELLE that a ventilator was the next step, I had a plan: I was Elle's primary doctor, and I was going to make a decision. Did I need permission from my colleagues to enact it? Technically, no. If Elle and I agreed to something, by all means we could go forward. Still, I wanted to proceed the right way. There's a fine line between an independent thinker and a poor team player, and I preferred not skating over it. I'd rather persuade my colleagues than blindside them.

I paged the pulmonologist on call. It was a different doctor from the one who did the bronchoscopy. "Another bronchoscopy would be low yield," he started, reading his colleague's note aloud.

"I'm actually calling with a different question," I said. "I want to start steroids for chemotherapy-induced pneumonitis. Can I get your blessing?"

I explained my literature search. I clarified why I was now less concerned about steroids exacerbating an infection. He listened. He agreed to take a look. A few hours later, I received a page with five beautiful words: "Agree to start empiric steroids."

With that endorsement, I knocked on Elle's door. "You're here late," she looked at me sympathetically. It was just after 7:00 p.m., and an empty tray showed remnants of a cafeteria dinner.

I got right to it. "I'd like to start some new medications, including steroids," I answered.

Elle looked alarmed. "Didn't you say no steroids because I'm infected?"

"I did," I admitted. "But now I'm more worried about not starting steroids."

It can be frightening for a patient to see her physicians do a one-eighty, but Elle listened with an open mind. She asked questions. She understood that things had changed and that a shifting analysis of risks and benefits was required. She wanted to breathe again, and so she agreed to try.

Alone at my computer, I typed orders for three new medications: high-dose steroids, an additional antifungal, and one more antibiotic to cover *Pneumocystis carinii* pneumonia, an infection that can colonize the lungs when steroids are suppressing the immune system. It was a lot. But while everything comes with risks, I didn't believe that any of these medications, alone or in combination, put her at more risk than she already was. This was my Hail Mary. I signed my orders.

That night the medications finished running through Elle's IV. When the overnight doctor came to check on her, her biggest complaint was that there was nothing good on TV.

WHEN I SAW ELLE THE NEXT MORNING, she was practically bouncing out of her bed. "I'm feeling much better!" she said.

Still we remained cautious. "Steroids make everyone feel better," the pulmonary attending reminded us. All objective measures of Elle's breathing, including how much oxygen she needed, hadn't improved. But they hadn't worsened either. A day passed, then another. Slowly, I weaned the oxygen we were delivering through her nasal cannula: ten liters went to eight, and eight liters went to six.

It took a few days, but it became undeniable. Elle's lungs were improving.

What happened next was equally fascinating. Medical culture gives doctors—correctly, I think—significant leeway to do what we feel is best in an emergency. We can all empathize with what it's like to make a call in such a situation, and we do not fault one another for urgently made decisions that don't end well. We recognize that we are on the same team, and we do not blame our coworkers for doing their best.

I learned from Elle Park that the same holds true for an unexpected happy ending. Buoyed by the positive payoff of a gamble gone well, history was immediately rewritten to reflect a unified front. The infectious diseases team approached me outside Elle's room. "It's a good thing we started steroids," the fellow who had advised not to start steroids said with a smile. "She's doing great!" I smiled back. We were a team, with the shared goal of seeing Elle get better.

Elle's story makes a case for investing in and rewarding generalists, who are responsible for the care of the entire patient and tend to be more accustomed to thinking beyond one organ system. It also makes a case for solid generalist training no matter a doctor's specialty. It justifies the time we spend in hospitals and clinics, caring for the young and the old along the spectrum of healthy to seriously ill and every iteration in between. Some doctors moan and groan their way through and breathe a sigh of relief when they finally settle into the niche of their chosen specialty, but the best doctors I've met don't. They hold onto their breadth as they develop depth. They don't overstep their expertise but understand that their expertise is just one piece of the puzzle.

We must also rethink the siloed mindsets that specialization can inculcate. It is unreasonable to expect every doctor not only to do a deep dive into their area of expertise but to maintain a thirty-thousand-foot view of a patient's full medical life. Yet to overcome the fragmented stories we tell ourselves, we must think actively about how to see the whole ones. To accomplish this, we have to be aware of the stories spun by other doctors, take proactive steps to consider whether they add up to a reasonable conclusion, and push ourselves to reconcile them if they don't. The empowering fact of the matter is that this doesn't take knowing the right answer off the bat. Sometimes it's as simple as raising a question. The status quo isn't working. Is there something we're missing?

Anyone can do this. Generalists can do this. Specialists, like the hematologist who pinpointed the significance of the CMV, can do this. Patients and loved ones can see when medical teams are working past one another and advocate for them to come together. Questioning whether all the pieces amass into a sensible whole does not threaten the health care dynamic but encourages us to see better by confronting our blind spots.

For Elle Park, the most radical act I performed was not disagreement with other doctors; it was suggesting that there was even a decision to be made. The radical act was deciding to decide.

BUT IN THE END, there was a narrative about Elle that I missed, too. My vantage point as Elle's doctor allowed me to tell myself a story about chemotherapy, invasive fungal infections, and pneumonitis. I neglected to see something else as a human being.

A month passed, and Elle's breathing continued to improve until she required no extra oxygen whatsoever. Her drenching fevers vanished. We gradually peeled off all antibiotics and antifungals and tapered her steroids to low doses. Our teams were united in the conclusion: this was a success story.

We were making plans for follow-up in the hematology clinic. Her blood counts were starting to recover, and she'd need another bone marrow biopsy to confirm that her leukemia was in remission.

A hematologist who rotated onto the case and who knew Elle from a previous hospitalization was skeptical. "Elle Park?" he said. "She hates doctors. And after this? She's not going to come back."

"She will," I said.

She didn't.

Elle missed one appointment and then another. The next time I rotated in clinic and was scheduled to see her, I eagerly pulled up her electronic chart only to find a trail of missed calls and unreturned voicemails. I sadly documented our visit together as a no-show. I realized that I had never seriously broached the subject of what comes after the hospitalization. I had taken for granted that curing Elle's leukemia, no matter how hard it would be, was a goal we shared.

In retrospect the clues to the contrary were there. Within the narrow walls of her hospital room, Elle told me she wanted to live. Yes, she wanted the steroids; she was willing to try anything that would help her breathe better. But it was more complicated than that. She was longing for home and anxious about anything that would keep her in the hospital longer. Even though she wanted to live, I didn't know what she wanted that life to look like or what additional trade-offs she'd be willing to make to get there.

One winter day—six months after I started her on steroids and treatment for a rare fungal infection and five months after we celebrated her discharge from the hospital—a nurse showed me an obituary published in a local newspaper. "Loving mother," it read. "Dedicated community servant." I learned that Elle passed away at home with family by her side. There was no mention of what she died from.

There is a lot I don't know. I don't know how she spent those months. I never found out if she made it to New York for Christmas. I wish I understood the calculus that led to her decision not to seek further treatment. I longed to know whether it was ultimately clear-eyed or whether she had wrestled with doubts.

One year later, I attended a medical conference that happened to be a few miles from where Elle had lived. That morning I hastily tapped the conference address into my GPS, and it dawned on me just where I was going. After attending a talk on molecular mechanisms of immune escape, I escaped. I got in my car and drove along a one-lane road, passing stretches of ranch houses and stopping when I found the beach Elle told me I had to visit.

As I sat on a log that smelled like seaweed, I pictured Elle here with her daughters. I imagined space for closure—time to say goodbye and I'm sorry and I love you. Elle's life didn't amount only to the number of years and months she lived. It included how the final chapters unfolded. While I don't know how Elle passed, I do know how she didn't. She wasn't in the hospital. She wasn't on a ventilator. Her family wasn't forced to gather amid the beeping monitors and hum of life support and make the most difficult choices imaginable.

It was windy, and flecks of sand whipped against my face. I took a deep breath and held the air in my lungs, appreciating the simple, incredible, life-sustaining ability to do so before I slowly let it out. I remembered Elle and I grieved her, but I had no regrets.

Chapter 9

Fixing Fragmentation Together

M Y FIRST WEEK AS A DOCTOR, I LEARNED ABOUT CHEESE. I was at an orientation at my new hospital, staring at a PowerPoint slide that depicted a model for how errors occur in complex systems such as health care. In 1990 a cognitive psychologist named James Reason published a book called *Human Error,* in which he proposed a now-famous metaphor for how these errors can occur. In the "Swiss cheese model," imagine several slices of Swiss cheese stacked back-to-back. Each slice represents a defense. Each hole represents potential for error. When multiple cheesy safeguards are in place, one hole by itself doesn't cause problems. But when all the holes align, disaster strikes.

Consider, we were told, how a wrong medication could be given to a patient. In this case, the slices of cheese—the defenses against it—could represent electronic alerts flagging an incorrect dosage, a pharmacist double-checking the medication before dispensing, or a nurse verifying a patient's name and date of birth. The holes could include a doctor's cognitive slip in ordering the wrong prescription or an electronic chart's failing to flag this slip once entered into the computer.

Scholars have poked holes in Reason's cheese holes since he published his ideas. The model has been criticized for being too simplistic and for portraying the escalation of error as a linear event, disregarding the back and forth that often occurs if a slip is noted.

(For example, a nurse who saw a suspicious order in the real world would likely call the doctor.) Others have pointed out that a safeguard introduced to prevent error in one place can unintentionally cause problems elsewhere. (I think of electronic alerts; too many can bombard doctors into accidentally clicking through the ones that matter.) Reason himself has acknowledged the model's limitations, giving a 2004 conference talk in France with the title "Is Swiss Cheese Past Its Sell-By Date?"

Yet more than thirty years after Reason introduced it and nearly a decade after I learned about it, the Swiss cheese model is still widely taught across health care fields because of its memorable simplicity and imagery. Acknowledging latent problems in the design of our system is a powerful message to make the system as a whole more resilient.

I found myself thinking about Swiss cheese again as I began cataloging different types of fragmentation in medicine. I imagined each hole: disparate electronic records that are not shared among doctors or with patients; clunky software that buries useful data; insurance barriers and scheduling restrictions that obstruct follow-up with a regular doctor; a medical culture that reacts to snapshots in time at the expense of the long term; a specialist's lens that loses sight of the bigger picture. Each of these holes is large, and none are mutually exclusive.

For a doctor, if your patient does poorly, it's always a good idea to retrace your steps and look for holes. But it doesn't necessarily mean you'll find them, just as a happy ending doesn't necessarily indicate a flawless performance. The complicated nature of our work means that untangling patchable holes from twists of fate is bound to be a messy and imperfect endeavor. But to make headway in improving health care, we must strive to be clear about the difference. Fixing fragmentation in health care requires teasing apart what we *don't* know because of preventable gaps from what we *can't* know because of radical uncertainty. And that means asking ourselves hard questions about what is in and out of our control—especially when all the obstacles of fragmentation present themselves at once.

THE STORY OF A WOMAN I'LL CALL Marisol Soares illustrates a perfect storm of fragmentation. Marisol didn't know it at the time, but she had two things growing inside her. When she became pregnant with her fourth child, she was overjoyed. But then odd things started to occur. She noticed she was bleeding into the toilet bowl after passing a bowel movement. She expected her pregnancy to make her gain weight as her other pregnancies had done, but the opposite was happening. By her second trimester, her maternity clothes were so baggy she didn't need them.

Marisol was thirty-three years old. She was healthy. Her first three pregnancies were easier on her than she anticipated and caused no medical complications. So she never saw the need to have a regular doctor. She spent her days working as the cashier in a family-owned shop. Health insurance was not something that came with the family business package.

Despite these factors, she was now concerned enough to seek medical care. She went to see an internal medicine doctor at an urgent care clinic and told him about the bleeding—sometimes just streaks, sometimes so much it turned the toilet bright red. "I just want to know I'm OK," she said. He looked at her pregnant belly, ordered no tests, and said she should come back if the bleeding persisted after she delivered.

But that was four months away. When a sharp ache in Marisol's lower abdomen began to accompany her bleeding, she sought a second opinion from a gastroenterologist. His opinion was similar to the first doctor's; he sent her away. When she continued to drop pounds, she sought a third opinion from an obstetrics nurse practitioner, who reassured her that the baby was doing fine and said to ask her primary care doctor—a person who did not exist for Marisol—about the blood in the toilet. Three different medical professionals dismissed her. Viewed through the narrowest of lenses, Marisol was a pregnant woman first, and no health care provider ventured past this lens. Further, because she lacked a regular doctor, no follow-up was arranged. Marisol was on her own.

From the outset, the holes were aligned for Marisol to slip through, and slip through she did. Months passed. A healthy baby grew in her uterus, while a few inches over, a tumor gnawed its way through her colon. As her baby formed eyes and ears and limbs, the tumor reached into nearby organs.

Eight weeks shy of her delivery date, she went to the emergency room. The dull ache she had grown accustomed to had turned into severe cramping. It must be labor, Marisol assumed. But an ultrasound followed by an MRI finally showed the truth.

The obstetrician called the gastroenterologist, who arranged for an immediate colonoscopy. A tube with a camera was inserted into her rectum, and to the gastroenterologist's horror, the camera displayed a mass that spanned the full diameter of a part of her colon. Biopsies proved that it was colon cancer.

Removing the cancer was urgent, but the baby had to come out first. The obstetrician induced labor, and Marisol gave birth seven weeks early. Then she and her newborn were split up. Baby Rafael went to the neonatal ICU, while Marisol was wheeled on a gurney to the oncology ward, where I was a senior resident at the time.

As a doctor and especially as an oncologist, I am careful to speak in a way that doesn't lay blame. Whenever I meet a patient with a new cancer diagnosis or someone who survived a cancer even decades earlier, they often ask me for an explanation. "How did I get this?" they wonder. Was it related to diet? Was it an exposure from my work? I try not to indulge in what-ifs. Cancer is a genetic mistake that causes uncontrolled replication of cells, I say.

For patients with current cancers, I explain in both current and future terms: This is where we are now. The tumor is here; it has spread this far; this is what we do next. I say these things because charting a plan forward is more productive than agonizing over what can't be changed.

In general, doctors also try not to play Monday-morning quarterback about the decisions of our colleagues. With the advantage of hindsight, it's easy to list what you would have done differently. As I listened to Marisol's backstory, I reminded myself that I hadn't been there. Maybe each doctor who saw Marisol during her pregnancy had ten-minute slots and dozens of patients left to see. They probably lacked adequate time or resources for a comprehensive evaluation because these are things we all could use more of.

But in Marisol's case, it was hard to maintain that narrative. I couldn't help but also imagine the individual choices that led to this point. I fantasized about going back in time, ordering a colonoscopy, and catching the tumor before it spread. Mostly I feared the road ahead. At that point, it wasn't yet clear just how deeply this cancer had invaded. It wasn't clear if those few months made the difference between a curable illness and a terminal one. The sadness of that possibility was almost too gut-wrenching to take.

The day after she delivered, I stood outside Marisol's hospital room door with a Portuguese interpreter and the medical intern on my team as we discussed what we would and wouldn't say. Records were being faxed. We were digging through the chart. Blood tests and scans were pending. There were still many unknowns, but it was time to meet.

We knocked on the door, and Marisol sat up in her hospital bed. We pulled up chairs and introduced ourselves as doctors on the oncology team. She pointed to two men sitting next to her: one was her boyfriend, Lucas, and the other was her older brother, Cris. We congratulated Marisol on the baby boy. We asked the baby's name. We asked the ages of her other children and how they felt about their new sibling. We tried to ease into the conversation that had brought us there, but I could see that Marisol wasn't having it. She was lying in a hospital bed in the oncology ward when she should have been going home with a newborn. There was nothing easy about this situation.

"I am sorry this is happening," I said next. "What have you heard about why you are here?"

"I have colon cancer," she answered in Portuguese. She had heard the likely diagnosis from the obstetrician who delivered Rafael and the definitive one from the gastroenterologist who performed the scope. Yet each had deferred discussing the details of what to do next.

I nodded and proceeded to review the information we had so far, emphasizing that we were still in the process of gathering data and that we would talk about prognosis when we learned more. I told her she would have a full body CT scan to determine if the cancer had spread to any distant places, like her liver or lungs. If it hadn't spread far away, we would make preparations to start chemotherapy. This would shrink the cancer's growth through the colon and nearby organs before a surgery could attempt to remove it.

Something I said was apparently news to her. "What organs?" she wanted to know.

I spoke slowly. "There appears to be cancer in the small bowel and the uterus." She looked at me, blinking. "It's also visible in the bladder."

A wail escaped her that remains seared in my memory. Then— "Am I going to die?"

No DOCTOR CAN MAKE IT to the end of medical training today without being able to answer this question. We are thankfully past the days when training neglected the so-called "softer" skills of being a doctor, such as communication, empathy, and ethical decision-making. Medical schools today have dedicated curricula on patient-doctor communication and on difficult conversations in particular. When I was a medical student, I remember practicing giving bad news. As I told my patient—who was really an actress—that the pain in her back was actually metastatic breast cancer and that it was incurable, an instructor watched from behind a two-way mirror. Afterward, the actress and instructor both gave me feedback on everything from my words to my body language. Later my training grew more creative, with videotaped interviews where I could go back and cringe at myself on demand.

Today hard conversations are a core part of what I do. I've developed an approach based on ideas I learned from the palliative care field. Establish emotional safety. Listen more than you talk. Look for the question behind the question. Don't overload with information. Validate the patient's emotions, and affirm you are on the same team, such as by saying, "I wish things were different." When discussing prognosis, give a range that includes the best-case, worst-case, and most likely scenarios. Address a Plan B: "We hope for the best but prepare for the worst." These tactics give me a foundation, but there is no template, and sometimes you don't know where the conversation will go. I've learned to follow my patients' cues.

I also know that questions like "Am I going to die?" and "How long do I have to live?" are fraught not only because of their emotional gravity but also because of unanticipated curveballs. I initially thought the challenge of these conversations hinged on communication: How can I convey highly emotional information with authenticity and kindness? How can I share hard truths without torpedoing hope? The implication in my training was that we doctors hold the truth; the hard part is deciding what to share and how to share it. But what if the truth isn't known? A full decade after I was praised for telling my fictive patient that her back pain was incurable cancer, I questioned that assumption. Questions about the details flooded my mind: Did a biopsy confirm it? Were there other sites of spread? Was the tumor genetically tested to see if novel medications could be tried? I knew it was just an exercise, but I found, amazingly, that I was less certain about the prognosis as a fully trained oncologist than I had been as a medical student.

Doctors, it turns out, are not very good at predicting how our patients will fare. One often-cited study from 2000 asked doctors how long they anticipated their terminally ill patients would survive. Only 20 percent were accurate (for everyone else who got it wrong, most overestimated survival, though the mistakes certainly spanned both directions). Moreover, the longer the doctor-patient relationship lasts, the more inaccurate the doctors' predictions, suggesting that close relationships can skew accurate prognostication. More recent studies have backed this. In one study, published in 2013, doctors were asked to predict how long patients with advanced cancer had; they were right only 56 percent of the time. Notably, these studies didn't look at how doctors *communicated* bad news; they homed in directly on doctors' beliefs.

Nothing drives this point home more than getting it wrong yourself. I once admitted to the cardiac ICU a ninety-year-old woman with advanced heart failure. A heart normally pumps at around 60 percent of its full capacity. Hers was at 10 percent. She had been in and out of the hospital over the last year with complications from heart failure, and these episodes were becoming more frequent. I started her on continuous infusions of medications to augment her heart function and to remove excess fluid. One night when I was on overnight call, her condition got worse. As her breathing quickened and she grew disoriented, I upgraded her oxygen support to a bilevel positive airway pressure mask that helped push air into her lungs. I checked blood test results every few hours that showed her carbon dioxide level rising and her oxygen falling. I tinkered with the drips running into her veins, but nothing worked. She had an advance directive clearly stating that she did not wish to be placed on a ventilator. It was a constellation of findings I thought I knew well: this is what dying looks like.

I called the cardiology attending, who thanked me for my efforts and agreed there was nothing more to do. That evening I spoke to her son. "I am concerned your mom will not survive the night," I told him. "If there is anyone else she would want to see, I recommend you call them now."

Over the next few hours, family members trickled in—three sons, some nieces and nephews, and grandchildren accompanied by stuffed animals. They set up chairs around her bedside, sometimes chatting and sometimes staying silent, sometimes holding her hand and sometimes giving her space. Eventually the sun came up. When I went to check on her, she had taken off her breathing mask and was slathering butter on a slice of toast.

"How are you?" I asked.

"I'm fine, dear," she answered. "And you?"

I was reluctant to face her son, wondering how he would react to the incorrectly dire picture I had painted. But no one regretted staying the night. It was a special time their family shared, renewing their focus on what mattered until she died peacefully at home three months later.

Knowing this unpredictability exists, how do we communicate honestly while acknowledging the uncertainty? One temptation is to be vague. I know other doctors—doctors I respect and admire—who dogmatically refuse to get into survival curves and stash away numbers when patients reach for them. The range is too large, they argue, and the ability to predict any individual's course teems with error. They know the same data that I do on how often doctors get the prognosis wrong, so they stay away. These are good doctors, motivated not by paternalistic impulses to obscure the truth but by a wealth of experience that tells them just how much we cannot predict.

However, obscuring doesn't feel quite right either. People deserve a chance to plan their lives and to create meaning as they conceive it, especially as time grows short. To do that, one must have a sense of how much is left. As Paul Kalanithi, the late Stanford neurosurgery resident who was diagnosed at the age of thirty-six with stage 4 lung cancer, wrote, "Now, instead of wondering why some patients persist in asking statistics questions, I began to wonder why physicians obfuscate when they have so much knowledge and experience. . . . The truth that you live one day at a time didn't help: What was I supposed to do with that day?"

When discussing prognosis, I have done it all. I have shared great detail out of a moral impulse that people deserve a chance to plan their lives and a sense of responsibility to use my knowledge to that end—and I have been wrong. I have been vague as a kind of truer honesty when appreciating the impossibility of predicting—and I have regretted withholding.

In the face of radical uncertainty, I have landed on an approach of radical honesty. "Let me tell you exactly what I'm thinking," I say. I ask patients how they prefer to hear information. Then I share what I know, with caveats: New facts will emerge. Twists are expected. We will take each decision as it comes. And when I have the gift of continuity with patients, I promise I will always be honest, based on the information we have and to the best of my ability.

Sharing bad news with caveats of medical uncertainty is challenging enough. What we aren't taught is how to convey the compounded uncertainty created by a fragmented health care system. I never learned to qualify "let's see what the CT scan shows" with "if I can access the records." I never learned to temper "we will wait and see" with "if I am able to see you in follow-up." When patients ask me if they are going to die, I do not say that it depends on whether we can sort through their electronic chart in time or whether we can come together as a team to reconcile specialists' differing narratives. It is my practice to be honest about uncertainty. But honesty about this? Conveying the deep failures of our fragmented system is next-level truth telling; I still lack the words to express this.

FOR THE NEXT FEW DAYS, our top priority was piecing together Marisol's story. Even within the same hospital system, the electronic charts on the pediatric side where Marisol delivered Rafael were disconnected from the adult wards a few hallways down. One doctor on our team took a trip to the children's hospital. However, without a log-in to the computer system there, she had to track down a busy doctor on the ob-gyn team to print a stack of paper records. Another doctor held two phones to her ears, waiting on hold with the lab to get biopsy results while trying to schedule Marisol for a port to administer chemotherapy. I worked on expediting full-body scans and ordered blood tests called tumor markers, only to discover that some of these test results were already in the records from the pediatric wing. As it had been with Michael Champion, our process was not perfect as we navigated the tension of collecting and collating data as quickly as possible without missing anything critical. We allowed ourselves some waste and repetition in the interest of accuracy without further delay.

One afternoon Marisol's heart rate jumped and stayed in the 150s. For days she expressed that she was terrified, but fear alone didn't account for such a big jump. My antennae went up, and a fever of 101.5 degrees Fahrenheit shortly after confirmed my suspicions. Her electronic chart raised a sepsis alert, and this time, unlike with Mitch Garter, the chart alerted us correctly. We ordered blood cultures, urine cultures, and a chest X-ray. We infused fluids and started broad IV antibiotics.

When the tests came back negative but the fevers persisted, we ordered a CT of her abdomen and pelvis. I scrolled through the images and saw what looked to be an abscess, a collection of infection, near the tumor. The most concerning image showed what appeared to be free air in the abdomen outside of the bowel—something that should never exist. It raised the possibility that part of her gut had ruptured.

In an instant, everything changed. The choice of what to do next was now deeply complicated. Antibiotics alone would not fix the anatomical calamity in Marisol's abdomen. Chemotherapy to treat the underlying colon cancer would suppress her immune system severely, emboldening the infection. Surgery to repair the hole was high risk while she was acutely septic.

But, as with Elle Park, inaction too was untenable. We had to find a way out, and now was the time for creativity. The choices are never simply chemo or surgery. We had to dig deeper. I had the idea to drain the abscess through a minimally invasive tube. If we drained the pus as the antibiotics simultaneously began to work, perhaps we could buy ourselves a safe window for chemotherapy. So we reviewed the case with a team of interventional radiologists. The tumor was in the way, they said. There was just no good path for tube insertion.

We examined Marisol's case from all angles, asking ourselves multiple questions: Can we get control of the infection another way? Are the antibiotics covering all possible culprits? What if we used a gentler type of chemotherapy that wouldn't cause so much immunosuppression?

The attending oncologist—I'll call her Linda—was developing a particular expertise in colon cancer and had a baby of her own at home. In all the time I've known her, her greatest strength has been her ability to recognize when she needs help. She suggested we call two other oncologists. Both had been in practice for decades. Both were respected experts in colorectal tumors nationally and internationally and had treated thousands of patients over their storied careers. Both were trusted mentors in our hospital.

One recommended surgery. The other said chemo.

We turned back to the surgery team. The chief resident balked, reiterating that a surgery now would carry serious risk of death. So the surgical team did exactly what we did—solicited more opinions. They projected Marisol's CT scans on a big screen while an experienced group of surgeons weighed in from around the room. Experts upon experts agreed: surgery could potentially patch the hole, but it wouldn't remove all the cancer.

Uncertainty was melting away, leaving in its place something much worse. As I watched Marisol shuttle between the oncology ward and the neonatal ICU to hold Rafael, I knew there was no way out. Marisol was going to die.

THE TRAGIC TURN OF EVENTS in Marisol's story meant that an evolution that often takes place over years was compressed into just a handful of days. As her future crystallized, our task had shifted— from conveying a range of possible futures to delivering news of the worst one.

We set up a meeting between Marisol, her boyfriend Lucas, her brother Cris, and all the doctors. There were eight doctors total, including representatives from oncology, surgery, and palliative care. We were an intimidating group even when a person is not hearing the worst news of her life. But each of us brought a perspective that contributed to the whole, and we were resolved to have this conversation as thoroughly and delicately as possible.

After we completed our introductions, I opened: "We are going to talk about some things today that may be difficult to hear." Marisol nodded, giving us permission to continue. We took turns speaking as we reviewed the cancer, the infection, and the initial plan for chemotherapy that was now off the table. We broached surgery as the only viable option, but just as we were getting into the details, she stopped us.

"Don't tell me!" she said. Her heart rate spiked. Her breaths were quick and shallow. Holding Lucas's hand with her right hand and gripping Cris's arm with her left, she looked around the room at the white coats and repeated something over and over in Portuguese. The interpreter couldn't hold back tears as she translated in a soft voice: "Please save my life! Please save me. Please save me. Please save me."

The next thing Marisol did was ask us to leave. She spent a few hours alone with her boyfriend and brother. Later that day, she said she was ready to hear more.

We somehow arranged for our large group to reconvene, and we shuffled back into her room. For the next hour, we discussed the risks and benefits of surgery. The surgeons explained that they would remove part of Marisol's colon and small bowel. This would leave her with a colostomy bag to pass stool through a stoma in her abdomen. They would also remove at least part of her bladder and possibly the whole thing. This would leave her with a pouch made out of intestine that would drain urine through another stoma. Her uterus would also be removed, meaning she could never carry another pregnancy.

It was possible she would not survive the surgery. It was possible she would die in the postoperative period. Another possibility was that she would survive both but endure a long recovery. We anticipated weeks to months of hospitalization followed by rehabilitation. During this time, she would be too sick to receive chemotherapy, and so the cancer would grow.

"The surgery will not cure the cancer," the attending surgeon emphasized.

At this point, Cris had begun weeping and couldn't speak more. Marisol stared at the floor. After a lot of questions from Lucas—

"Do we have to decide now? Can a second surgery be done later to get the cancer?"—they were beginning to understand. With her hands locked together, not looking up from the ground, Marisol finally asked in a whisper, "Is there any way I will survive?"

There was silence for a moment. "I don't think so," the surgeon responded.

The palliative care doctor was quick to clarify. Incurable cancer did not mean incurable suffering. We had good medications to relieve symptoms like pain and nausea and resources that would help with caregiving at home.

At this point, the palliative care doctor also clarified that there was a choice. If Marisol decided against surgery, we would continue to give antibiotics. Marisol would be allowed to spend time with her baby and her family, knowing that this time would be short. She would die from infection or its complications within days, weeks at best.

Lucas asked how much more time Marisol would get with the surgery. This time Linda committed to an answer: "The best-case scenario is a year and a half."

Everyone said nothing for a long time. When Marisol finally spoke, she was resolute. "If the surgery is the only way to spend more time with my family, I want you to do it." Then she got out of bed, lunged toward a trash can, and dry-heaved into it.

To THIS DAY, I recall that conversation as one of the most difficult of my career. I include the middle-aged woman who punched the air and cursed me out after I told her that more chemotherapy for her stage 4 sarcoma would not help her live longer or better. I include the forty-two-year-old who, when her lung cancer progressed, told us with clear-eyed confidence that she was ready to die, as her husband and parents screamed, cried, and tried to change her mind with every argument they had. I include the undocumented man who, alone and two thousand miles from his family, begged me to end his life when a tumor in his spinal cord paralyzed him from the neck down.

As heart-wrenching as our conversation with Marisol and her loved ones was, it went as well as it could have given the circumstances. By all measures, we offered Marisol choices. We respected *how* she wanted to hear bad news and honored her wishes to give her time alone first. We gave a range of estimates that included the best-case, worst-case, and most likely scenarios. We expressed empathy while remaining consistent in our messaging.

Fragmented health care has many harmful consequences, from incubating medical errors to burdening patients and providers with logistical gymnastics. In our conversation with Marisol, we narrowly escaped yet another: the repetition of bad news. In 2017 the pediatric oncologist and bioethicist Amy Caruso Brown wrote a powerful account showing how this can happen, using the example of her teenaged patient "K," who was told the devastating news that her leukemia was back. "It is a truism in medicine that patients often hear something quite different from what physicians think they have said," Caruso Brown wrote. "Of course, the opposite is also true. I doubt any of the physicians were aware that, after K's last relapse, her family had been told she was going to die 47 separate times in 72 hours—nor that K's mother was counting."

Caruso Brown's story was familiar. As an oncology fellow, I once admitted a soft-spoken man in his seventies to the hospital for a small bowel obstruction. The obstruction, which caused severe nausea, vomiting, and constipation, was caused by the growth of his advanced pancreatic cancer. We inserted a nasogastric tube to relieve his bloating and infused plenty of fluids through his IV. Within a few days, the obstruction improved. While he was hospitalized, he had a few other problems that we fine-tuned, including an arrhythmia that required adjusting his pacemaker settings.

I stood outside his room with the cardiologist, who took one look at the chart and sighed.

"I could adjust the pacemaker," he said, "but this patient is *dying*. That's what we need to tell him."

I couldn't let that happen. "He knows," I answered.

It was a recurring pattern. I heard it from everyone: the nurse, the social worker, the case manager, the intern, the surgical resident. *We have to tell him.* A fragmented team working in silos meant that each provider had no idea what anyone else said, much less what the patient had been told. Thinking about the big picture is always a good idea, but in this case, my patient was already deep into these talks with his regular doctor. It felt less like being honest about prognosis and more like browbeating someone about his impending doom.

When wrestling with competing interests—a person needs to know his prognosis to plan, and a person benefits from maintaining hope—is there a tightrope that physicians can really walk? Is there a way to avoid the dual traps of dangling false hope and bulldozing with bad news?

An oncologist named Paul Helft argues that there is. He published an article asserting that although "common wisdom holds that [doctors] should give accurate and honest prognostic information to patients at all times," he favors a communication tactic that "allows the cold, hard facts to come out over time." This "necessary collusion," as he calls it, is not dishonest. Quite the contrary—by taking a stepwise approach to doling out bad news, not only does someone's prognosis become clearer, but patients become more receptive to hearing it.

Helft's perspective takes for granted two things we don't always get. The first is continuity—that the same doctor will be able to dole out news with a patient. The second is time. While the approach can work for illnesses that progress as a series of losses, it's less applicable in cases of sudden, unexpected decline.

Still, whenever possible, the approach of spooning out bad news speaks to me because it is a framework for honesty within the confines of uncertainty. As a person's medical reality takes shape, she will be able to process, adjust her expectations, and take stock of what matters most. People will do this differently. Some will prepare wills and prioritize getting their finances in order. Some will spend all their waking hours with people they love. Some will fight and cry and rage against the dying of the light until they take their final breath. Our job as doctors is not to dictate the response but to give people an opportunity to react on their own terms.

OVER THE NEXT FEW DAYS, Marisol did just that. After our group conversation, Marisol decided there were some things she wanted to do. Her three other children were brought to the hospital and spent full days running through the hospital hallways, sitting on their mom's lap, and making silly faces at their new brother.

The day of the surgery, Marisol calmly signed the consent forms. She was at peace, she said. She accepted whatever was intended for her as the operating room was prepped and she slipped on her blue surgical cap and booties.

The surgeons went to work. It was an enormous, intricate, and dangerous operation. Colorectal surgeons, urologists, and gynecologic oncologists crowded around the operating table. They patched the hole and removed one organ after another as planned. The scope of the cancer was fully apparent, and the surgeons took extreme care to manage blood loss along the way.

In the recovery room, Marisol awoke and looked around. She had a breathing tube down her throat and drains protruding from her abdomen, but she was alive.

It would have been easy to celebrate, but now was not the time to get lax. We were up against the usual obstacles: Marisol, like

Burt Klein, was subject to doctors' long hours and a rotating cast in the ICU. With three teams of doctors (ICU, surgery, and oncology), we had to be extra careful not to talk past one another and lose sight of the whole. Finally, I worried that any mistaken reaction to a snapshot like in my father's case could postpone the long-term plan that we had no wiggle room to delay: getting her well enough to start chemotherapy.

As we visited her each morning, I gave pep talks to the rotating ICU residents. We were the gatekeepers to that extra year and a half of life with Rafael and her other children that Marisol prized. We had to be proactive, and we had to be vigilant. Over the next few days, we removed her breathing tube and catheters as soon as they were no longer needed. We gave her blood thinners and set compression devices to squeeze her legs to prevent clots. A subtle spike in her white blood cell count prompted us to order immediate tests, and we treated a new bacterial infection coursing through her bloodstream with antibiotics. Her nutrition was poor, and so we supplemented her diet with protein and carefully replenished electrolytes. We took it all seriously: constipation, infection, nutrition, pain control, mobility, mental health, and more. We knew that any complication could not only snowball medically but would delay her receiving chemotherapy. There could be no lingering because lingering meant more time for the cancer to grow unchecked.

Because we had a big-picture view of her timeline, our oncology team began planning for the next steps well before she was medically ready. The chemotherapy we wanted to give would involve infusing a three-drug cocktail every two weeks, monitoring her blood work, managing side effects, and adjusting her medications as needed. The entire course of treatment would take six months. It would cause hair loss, painful mouth sores, nausea, fatigue, and possible numbness in her fingers and toes. I was reminded of Jin Wong; everything now hinged on follow-up. Marisol needed medications and tests, but what she needed most was a doctor to oversee them. Because her hospitalization was considered an emergency, her lack of health insurance could not be used to turn her away. Everything that came next, however, would not be considered an emergency by our health care system's standards. Marisol had a team of doctors in the hospital, but who would be her doctor once she left?

Meeting after meeting with our case manager identified a solution: an angel of an oncologist who worked in a safety net hospital about an hour east. This easily could have gone a different way; I thought of my relentless phone calls to doctors who couldn't accept Jin. But this oncologist had expertise in colon cancer—a disease far more common than Jin's acute myeloid leukemia—and agreed to take on Marisol. We went to work. We wrote up thorough discharge summaries and faxed them. We called over and had a detailed conversation with the oncologist to highlight the important parts of Marisol's plan that even comprehensive records might obscure.

I was relieved that we found a solution to yet another one of Marisol's problems. But deep down I remained worried. Marisol still needed weeks of rehabilitation before the chemotherapy could start, and a lot could fall through in that time. Even if she were able to proceed, the chemotherapy would tether her to appointments and induce an array of side effects that would hamper her quality of life. The drugs could cause a serious, life-threatening complication as she was recovering from major surgery. The cancer could grow back quickly anyway. Marisol was finally feeling motivated, though, and who was I to quash it? She dressed and packed her bags. Before discharging her from the hospital, I wished her luck. There was nothing left to do but hope.

IT IS A WELL-KNOWN STATISTIC that one-quarter of Medicare spending in the United States occurs in the last year of life. This fact is bemoaned by policymakers and the public alike because it is usually interpreted as waste. Most package it as a problem of doctors overtreating at the end of life due to all sorts of warped incentives, such as financial gain, communication failure, or self-delusion. But this narrative never sat right with me. I think of all the times I've been called down to the emergency room, started treatment on an extremely sick patient—and waited. Some patients got better; some didn't. Of course the last year of life is when spending is high. Patients are sick, and the goal is to prevent dying and prolong meaningful life. It's not like it's futile from the start. Plus, could anyone argue that the extra year and a half we tried to give thirty-three-year-old Marisol with her four children including a new baby was *futile*?

In 2018 three economists and an emergency doctor debunked the waste theory with data. Using a machine-learning model, they showed that less than 5 percent of spending is on patients with a predicted mortality above 50 percent. The rest is spent not on those who are clearly dying but on those who are sick. As the researchers put it, "These common interpretations of end-of-life spending flirt with a statistical fallacy: those who end up dying are not the same as those who were sure to die." It's easier to blame doctors for hiding the truth than to reckon with the knowledge that doctors often don't know.

As a society, we have spent enormous effort and sums of money trying to find ways around medical uncertainty. Researchers develop prediction models, and we plug numbers into them to calculate our destiny. Patients ask me if they should tattoo "do not resuscitate" on their bodies. We want to pin down our wishes before it's too late. This is admirable, but it usually isn't realistic. Planning can help guide us, but nailing down specifics is rooted in fantasy. When I ask patients what they want near the end, most people say remarkably similar things. They don't want invasive or heroic efforts. They don't want to feel pain. They want comfort and peace. Medically, these are all very doable. But the deeper question gnaws: when is the end? And if we doctors can't always make this call, how can we expect anyone else to?

In reality, no matter how much one prepares, there will often be a moment when a decision must be made. A man with advanced lung cancer presents with shortness of breath and hypoxia, and the CT scan shows possible pneumonia. Is this a treatable setback with antibiotics and intubation, or is this how he dies? A woman with severe heart failure develops critically low blood pressure. Do you recommend going to the ICU, placing a central line, and starting vasopressors in the hopes of finding something reversible? An older man who has endured a long list of medical complications has an abdominal perforation. Do you offer to take him to the operating room and close the hole, or is this his final complication?

These are the moments someone must choose: yes, now, this is it, stop. We navigate this moment in different ways. Loved ones ask the doctor, what is the prognosis? Doctors defer to the patient or her family: what would she want? The hard truth is that uncertainty can persist right up until the end. Years of being called in and guiding so many patients through these instances—rapidly assessing the landscape, sometimes offering choices and sometimes deciding for patients when I sense they need it—I do not believe there is a way to get comfortable with the final branch point. The best we can strive for is making decisions we can stand by.

Today there is an idea in medicine that defines courage by knowing when to stop. This is no doubt a backlash to a long-entrenched culture that viewed a doctor's job as extending life at all costs, with the quality of that life never given more than a fleeting thought. It was correct and necessary to reevaluate the harm medicine could do by pushing too hard. But I worry about overcorrecting.

I believe true courage in medicine is addressing the situation at hand. It is examining all the details before making life-altering decisions. It is listening to what a patient wants without projecting what she should want and respecting those wishes even if—and especially when—they change over time. Sometimes, after dotting every i and crossing every t, the right choice is aggressive medical treatment. Sometimes it is letting go. Neither is the more heroic path. Guiding patients through the ups and downs of medicine takes an abundance of experience and intuition, and we still get it wrong sometimes. But we can do this without using clichéd battle metaphors that glamorize fighting or clobbering patients with the grimness of their prognoses. We can do this with humility, openness to a changing narrative, and ongoing conversation.

I USUALLY KEEP A LIST OF PATIENTS I want to check on after they leave the hospital. But after we discharged Marisol, I couldn't put her on any list. It was too personal. I was too invested. I knew what the outcome would be, and I didn't want to see it.

I never forgot her, though. I thought about her when I met patients, especially young women, who had been dismissed by other doctors. I vowed to be the change as I listened to them, diagnosed them, and treated them. I committed to communicating with compassion and honesty, even as uncertainty was the constant cloud under which I worked. I needed to be a part of the system that did better.

One day, three years later, I was rotating in the oncology clinic with Linda and looked at the schedule. Was it possible? It had to be someone with the same name. Could it really be?

It was. By this time, Marisol had finished chemotherapy. Her hair had regrown. Her mouth sores were healed. She gained back the weight she had lost. Rafael, now three, was there too, defying instructions not to touch the medical equipment. He hugged his mom's leg as plans were made to follow up in six months.

I learned that after Marisol finished chemotherapy, she enrolled in a new insurance plan, which allowed her to return to our clinics. Linda happened to be off the hospital wards and accepting new patients into her growing practice. With that kind of continuity rare, she eagerly accepted Marisol. Linda became Marisol's regular doctor, and Marisol became Linda's regular patient.

The chemotherapy Marisol received was meant to keep the cancer from growing, but it did more than that. At the end of it, she underwent a CT scan that showed no signs of cancer. One year later, and then two years later, scans showed the same.

The line between remission and cure is a blurry one. Remission means that the tests we have detect no signs of cancer, but we worry about microscopic disease that will allow the cancer to come back. When remission stretches out long enough, eventually we are comfortable using that desired word, cured—meaning the cancer is gone forever. But when can we say a patient is cured? After five years? After ten years? It is a hazy boundary, and many people with cancer are forced to live somewhere in between. What I can say is that Marisol reached a point where she stopped thinking about just surviving and started focusing on living.

What Marisol went through changed her. When I saw her in the clinic, the terrified woman who pleaded with us to save her life was gone. In her place was someone who reminded me of Sarah Leary: she asked detailed questions and was meticulously on top of her paperwork, prescriptions, and tests. The rite of passage was familiar. I know all too well the transformation from trusting the health care system, to having the epiphany that the burden is yours, to questioning and double-checking everything. Marisol and I share a mindset of constant vigilance.

But I must admit something. To this day, I find it hard to wrap my mind around how Marisol survived. Knowing intellectually that doctors are not good at predicting did little to cushion the shock of seeing her calmly filling out a form three years after we gave her a best-case scenario of one and a half years.

Patients like Marisol are the ones I will always remember. They humble me and make clear medicine's limitations to control outcomes. They are walking, breathing reminders of just how much we don't know and may never know.

It's an important lesson to learn. As a doctor, I see a lot of death. I witness a lot of suffering. Knowing that we cannot control everything protects us from self-blame when the patients we care about do not do well. Doctors already face depression and anxiety at extremely high levels. That's what happens when our decisions can cost someone a colon or a life. Kindness within our profession means recognizing that despite our best efforts, some things are out of our hands.

And yet, caring for so many patients over my years in practice, I have also seen just how much we can tip the scales. This is due not just to cutting-edge medicine but to a steadfast commitment to the totality of a patient's story. When facing the perfect storm of fragmentation Marisol's case presented, we fought to piece together the whole. When confronting an array of Swiss cheese holes, we plugged them with diligence, creativity, and persistence. Did our efforts guarantee Marisol's happy conclusion? Not alone they didn't. But could any slipup all but have ensured the opposite outcome? It pains me to imagine what would have happened had we not connected with the local oncologist who oversaw six months of chemotherapy; or if Marisol's biopsy records disappeared from the children's hospital; or if even a single complication in the ICU that resulted from rotating physicians working long shifts let her slip outside of the window for a cure.

These things were not simply possible; they were within a hair's breadth. And if one oversight did occur, we could say medicine is uncertain. We could say that Marisol Soares had an awful prognosis from the start. We could say that she had a terrible cancer. These narratives would all be true. But they also wouldn't be quite right.

The inevitability of medical uncertainty, to me, is a clarion call to fight all *other* kinds of uncertainty within health care. That means naming and defining fragmentation as the central issue it is. Making this distinction matters so deeply because fragmentation in health care is not inevitable. It is not a by-product of the complicated nature of human beings. It is by design, it is a product of choices, and it can be changed. Fixing it involves choices, too.

Here are some solutions we can choose. We can connect electronic records between doctors and hospitals. We can release data transparently to the very patients they involve. We can lean on technology to organize patient data in a safer, less error-prone way. We can restructure reimbursement to incentivize follow-up as the life-saving care it is. We can eradicate twenty-eight-hour shifts that fracture the care of critically ill patients and instead construct schedules to maximize relationships. We can invest more federal spending in primary care. We can change medical culture to reward zooming out past the moment or the body part to view the patient's full story.

Spending my life grappling with hard questions gives me purpose. Whenever a patient asks me, "Am I going to die?" it is a chance to enter gray zones with humility. Whenever someone asks me, "How long do I have to live?" I strive to convey uncertainty with compassion and authenticity.

After I watched Rafael hug his mother's leg, I walked out of the cancer center. It was rush hour, and I blended in with a crowd of white coats and scrubs shuffling alongside me. I thought about Marisol and Rafael and uncertainty. I thought about how time is borrowed for all of us and how to make the most of what we have. As I walked to the parking lot, I pulled my phone out of my white coat pocket. I tapped my parents' number and smiled at the sound of their voices.

"Work's good," I said. "How are you?"

The Full Story:
A Patient's Checklist

In our fragmented medical system, you are the only guaranteed source of continuity in your own care. Here are some things it is helpful to have on hand.

Personal Info

- Name:
- Date of birth:
- Phone number:
- Address:
- Emergency contact:
- Height, weight:
- Blood type:

Care Team

- My primary doctor:
- My specialist doctors:
- My other providers (e.g., mental health therapist or nutritionist):
- My health insurance carrier:

Chief Complaint

- I am here today because (e.g., "My chest hurts"):
- This has been going on for (e.g., "a few months"):
- The problem feels better when (e.g., "I take two extra-strength Tylenols"):
- The problem gets worse when (e.g., "I lie flat at night"):

Medical History

- Medical conditions (e.g., diabetes, cancer, heart disease, arthritis):
- Surgeries (when, where):
- Hospitalizations (when, where, and reason):
- Past treatments (e.g., chemotherapy, radiation therapy):

Medications

- Prescription medications (name, dosage, and how often I take):
- Over-the-counter medications:
- Other supplements, such as vitamins or herbs:
- Pharmacy where I pick up medications:

Allergies

- Allergies to medications:
- Allergies to anything else a doctor may give (e.g., IV contrast):
- What happens during an allergic reaction (e.g., "I get itchy"):

Immunizations

- Vaccines in the last ten years:

Tests

- Blood tests done recently:
- Imaging (e.g., X-rays, ultrasound):
- Pathology results (e.g., Pap smear, biopsy):
- Procedures (e.g., stress test, colonoscopy):

Health Habits

- Alcohol (how many drinks per week):
- Tobacco (how many packs a day and for how many years total):
- Drugs (what kind and how they are taken):
- My exercise routine:
- My diet:
- My sleep:
- My mental health:

Family History

- Medical conditions in first-degree relatives (parents, siblings, and children):

My Wishes

- Do I have an advance directive indicating my wishes in the case of a medical emergency?
- What does it say?
- Durable power of attorney (this names the one person I'd like to make medical decisions on my behalf if I cannot):

Acknowledgments

THIS BOOK EXISTS THANKS TO MY PATIENTS. TO THOSE WHOSE lives inspired these pages and the countless others I've had the privilege to treat, you are the reason I wrote this. I am grateful to all the patients who trusted me to be their doctor, even while the brokenness of our health care system is the air we breathe. I deeply thank Michael and Leah Champion, who bravely allowed me to use their real names in what became this book's origin story. I hope I did you justice.

I came to Stanford Medicine in 2015 to begin my work as a doctor. I never left. Stanford Medicine has been my academic home and community of friends. I fully believe I am the doctor I am today thanks to brilliant and unfailingly moral mentors and colleagues, too many to list here, who have been inspirational and aspirational. I thank the leadership of my medical center and division who have supported my medical journalism for years, including the writing of this book.

When I first envisioned the idea for this book, I called my literary agent, William Callahan. I remember pacing the floor as we hashed out where the book had potential and where it could go even further. I thank him for waiting patiently as I wrote a book proposal and for helping me navigate the publishing world to see it through.

My editor at W. W. Norton, Jessica Yao, has played an extraordinary role in shaping this work. She has balanced steady praise with an expert ability to point out my jargon and help me see my blind spots. She possesses a big-picture focus that every writer dreams of and has kept me on track. Quynh Do read and commented on my proposal and the first third of this manuscript. Both have made this book better in every way. I thank the rest of my team at Norton, Annabel Brazaitis, Pat Wieland, Robert Byrne, Julia Druskin, Sarahmay Wilkinson, Yang Kim, Meredith McGinnis, and Gabrielle Nugent, for their work in transforming a document on my laptop into a book out in the world.

I am grateful to my fact-checker, Andy Young, who combed through this book with a red pen (literally, I learned, as I heard papers flipping on our phone calls), indefatigable spirit, and good humor. He reinterviewed my sources and confirmed the statistics cited in this book.

Parts of this book were adapted from prior writing and have benefited from the wisdom of previous editors. I thank Tom Zeller, Brooke Borel, and Jane Roberts at *Undark Magazine* for bringing to publication a version of this book's first chapter. When I first pitched the story of fragmented medical records to Tom Zeller, I remember his words on the phone to "muscle it." Those words have stayed with me and pushed me to go deeper, report more, and think harder throughout the entire process of writing this book. The story of my father's illness was expanded from an article I published in *Health Affairs*, where my editor Jessica Bylander was instrumental in helping me hone my ideas and my prose. Ideas were also adapted from pieces I wrote at MDedge, where Mary Ellen Schneider and others supported my writing.

I count myself lucky that my sister, Dr. Shara Yurkiewicz, also happens to be my closest confidant and trusted sounding board. Many ideas in this book have come from our conversations over the years as we moved forward in our medical careers at the same time. I also thank Shara for reading early excerpts, where her editorial acumen was as insightful as everything else she brings to this world.

My husband, Andrew Esensten, has been by my side even when all my waking hours were devoted to medicine and writing. He has steadied me through my ups and downs, cheered me when my endurance faltered, and expertly distracted me when I needed to pause. He, too, read and commented on an early draft. I thank him for the feedback that has enriched my work and his presence that has enriched my life.

I would be remiss if I didn't thank the donors of the Palo Alto public park benches, who unknowingly gave me my wonderful weekend office space to write so many of these pages. Fresh air, beautiful scenery, and the confused looks of passing hikers became just the right motivation to complete this work.

Finally, I owe everything else to my parents, Jack and Shelley Yurkiewicz. Since I could crawl, they have supported my ambitions with a seriousness, respect, and love that every child deserves. They have role-modeled a goodness that has informed my life as a doctor, author, and human being. On top of everything, my parents gave me their blessing to write of our family's most painful time with the hope that my words can make a difference for others. Since I began writing, my father has kept a master list of every article I wrote and every interview I did with unwavering pride in being my "assistant." Dad, we can add this book to the list; I dedicate it to you and Mom.

Notes on Sources

Introduction

xiii **doctors spend two hours:** Christine Sinsky et al., "Allocation of Physician Time in Ambulatory Practice: A Time and Motion Study in Four Specialties," *Annals of Internal Medicine* 165, no. 11 (2016): 753–60.

xiii **half of doctors report burnout:** Medscape, "Physician Burnout and Depression Report," 2022, https://www.medscape.com/slideshow/2022-lifestyle-burnout-6014664#1.

Chapter 1: Paper Trails

6 **only 40 percent of hospitals:** Office of the National Coordinator for Health Information Technology, U.S. Department of Health and Human Services, "Interoperability among U.S. Non-Federal Acute Care Hospitals in 2015," ONC Data Brief, no. 36, May 2016.

6 **30 percent of skilled nursing facilities:** Office of the National Coordinator for Health Information Technology, U.S. Department of Health and Human Services, "Electronic Health Record Adoption and Interoperability among U.S. Skilled Nursing Facilities in 2016," ONC Data Brief, no. 39, September 2017.

6 **55 percent of hospitals:** Office of the National Coordinator for Health Information Technology, U.S. Department of Health and Human Services, "Use of Certified Health IT and Methods to Enable Interoperability by U.S. Non-Federal Acute Care Hospitals, 2019," ONC Data Brief, no. 54, February 2021.

8 **"We need to get them blended":** Karen DeSalvo, interview by Ilana Yurkiewicz, February 17, 2018.

9   **"Doctors, nurses, physician assistants":** Lucia Savage, interview by Ilana Yurkiewicz, March 1, 2018.

9   **"they're frustrated":** Mark Savage, interview by Ilana Yurkiewicz, February 21, 2018.

9   **A 2014 survey:** National Partnership for Women and Families, "Engaging Patients and Families: How Consumers Value and Use Health IT," December 2014, Washington, DC, https://www .nationalpartnership.org/our-work/resources/health-care/digital -health/archive/engaging-patients-and-families.pdf.

11   **In an article covering Google Health's launch:** Steve Lohr, "Google Offers Personal Health Records on the Web," *New York Times*, May 20, 2008.

11   **patients had not been notified:** Rob Copeland, "Google's 'Project Nightingale' Gathers Personal Health Data on Millions of Americans," *Wall Street Journal*, November 11, 2019.

11   **an anonymous whistleblower:** Anonymous, "I'm the Google Whistleblower: The Medical Data of Millions of Americans Is at Risk," *Guardian*, November 14, 2019.

12   **headline from *Wired*:** Gregory Barber and Megan Molteni, "Google Is Slurping Up Health Data—and It Looks Totally Legal," *Wired*, November 11, 2019.

12   **The *Atlantic* wrote:** Sidney Fussell, "Google's Totally Creepy, Totally Legal Health-Data Harvesting," *Atlantic*, November 14, 2019.

12   **CBS News announced:** Megan Cerullo, "Google Reportedly Mining Millions of Americans' Personal Health Data," CBS News, November 11, 2019.

12   **responded in a blog post:** David Feinberg, "Tools to Help Health-care Providers Deliver Better Care" (blog), November 20, 2019, https://blog.google/technology/health/google-health-provider -tools-launch/.

12   **sent a letter to Ascension CEO:** Letter from Senators Elizabeth Warren, Richard Blumenthal, and Bill Cassidy to Mr. Joseph R. Impicciche, President and Chief Executive Officer, Ascension, March 2, 2020, https://www.warren.senate.gov/imo/ media/doc/2020.03.02%20Letter%20to%20Ascension%20re%20 Project%20Nightingale%20Partnership.pdf.

17   **between 44,000 and 98,000 people:** Institute of Medicine, *To Err Is Human: Building a Safer Health System*, ed. Linda T. Kohn, Janet M. Corrigan, and Molla S. Donaldson (Washington, DC: National Academies Press, 2000).

17   **medical errors remain:** B. A. Rodwin et al., "Rate of Preventable Mortality in Hospitalized Patients: A Systematic Review and

Meta-analysis," *Journal of General Internal Medicine* 35, no. 7 (2020): 2099–106.

17 **they are largely ineffective:** Joint Commission, "Transitions of Care: The Need for a More Effective Approach to Continuing Patient Care," 2012, Oakbrook Terrace, IL.

17 **nearly 20 percent:** A. J. Forster et al., "The Incidence and Severity of Adverse Events Affecting Patients after Discharge from the Hospital," *Annals of Internal Medicine* 138, no. 3 (2003): 161–67.

17 **at least one discrepancy:** P. L. Cornish et al., "Unintended Medication Discrepancies at the Time of Hospital Admission," *Archives of Internal Medicine* 165, no. 4 (2005): 424–29.

17 **surveyed the resident physicians:** Marta Almli, unpublished data, email communication, September 2, 2018.

18 **when emergency rooms shared files:** E. J. Lammers, J. Adler-Milstein, and K. E. Kocher, "Does Health Information Exchange Reduce Redundant Imaging? Evidence from Emergency Departments," *Medical Care* 52, no. 3 (2014): 227–34.

18 **Another study, this one from Israel:** O. Ben-Assuli, I. Shabtai, and M. Leshno, "The Impact of EHR and HIE on Reducing Avoidable Admissions: Controlling Main Differential Diagnoses," *BMC Medical Informatics and Decision Making* 13, no. 49 (2013): https://doi.org/10.1186/1472-6947-13-49.

Chapter 2: Who Owns the Story?

27 **In twenty-one states:** Health Information and the Law, "Who Owns Medical Records: 50 State Comparison," last updated August 20, 2015, http://www.healthinfolaw.org/comparative-analysis/who-owns-medical-records-50-state-comparison.

27 **right to inspect and receive:** Health Insurance Portability and Accountability Act (HIPAA) of 1996, Pub. L. No. 104-191, 100 Stat. 2548, https://www.govinfo.gov/app/details/PLAW-104publ191.

27 **"If I were a patient":** Carolyn Lye, interview by Ilana Yurkiewicz, October 2, 2020.

29 **Lye would pose:** C. T. Lye et al., "Assessment of US Hospital Compliance with Regulations for Patients' Requests for Medical Records," *JAMA Network Open* 1, no. 6 (2018): e183014.

29 **how patients receive radiology results:** C. T. Lye et al., "Evaluation of the Patient Request Process for Radiology Imaging in U.S. Hospitals," *Radiology* 292, no. 2 (2019): 409–13.

33   **launched a small pilot:** T. Delbanco et al., "Inviting Patients to Read Their Doctors' Notes: A Quasi-Experimental Study and a Look Ahead," *Annals of Internal Medicine* 157, no. 7 (2012): 461–70.

33   **"We . . . don't deal very well with change":** Tom Delbanco, interview by Ilana Yurkiewicz, October 6, 2020.

Chapter 3: Making Computers Work for Us

50   **"Imagine going to a car rental place":** Mark Savage, interview by Ilana Yurkiewicz, February 21, 2018.

55   **nearly three million medical notes:** A. Rule et al., "Length and Redundancy of Outpatient Progress Notes across a Decade at an Academic Medical Center," *JAMA Network Open* 4, no. 7 (2021): e2115334.

55   **ordering Tylenol:** R. M. Ratwani et al., "A Usability and Safety Analysis of Electronic Health Records: A Multi-Center Study," *Journal of the American Medical Informatics Association* 25, no. 9 (2018): 1197–201.

56   **can approach four thousand:** R. G. Hill Jr., L. M. Sears, and S. W. Melanson, "4000 Clicks: A Productivity Analysis of Electronic Medical Records in a Community Hospital ED," *American Journal of Emergency Medicine* 31, no. 11 (2013): 1591–94.

56   **the size of their pupils:** S. Khairat et al., "Association of Electronic Health Record Use with Physician Fatigue and Efficiency," *JAMA Network Open* 3, no. 6 (2020): e207385.

57   **A poll by Stanford Medicine researchers:** Stanford Medicine, "How Doctors Feel about Electronic Health Records," National Physician Poll by the Harris Poll, Stanford University, Stanford, CA, 2018.

59   **examined 248 malpractice cases:** M. L. Graber et al., "Electronic Health Record-Related Events in Medical Malpractice Claims," *Journal of Patient Safety* 15, no. 2 (2019): 77–85.

60   **personally had missed abnormal findings:** H. Singh et al., "Information Overload and Missed Test Results in EHR-Based Settings," *JAMA Internal Medicine* 173, no. 8 (2013): 702–4.

63   **"I was bright-eyed and ambitious":** Devin Horton, interview by Ilana Yurkiewicz, December 21, 2020.

Chapter 4: Are You My Doctor?

86   **nearly one in ten:** A. J. Singer, H. C. Thode, and J. M. Pines, "US Emergency Department Visits and Hospital Discharges among

Uninsured Patients before and after Implementation of the Affordable Care Act," *JAMA Network Open* 2, no. 4 (2019): e192662.

95   **defined having a primary doctor:** D. M. Levine, B. E. Landon, and J. A. Linder, "Quality and Experience of Outpatient Care in the United States for Adults with or without Primary Care," *JAMA Internal Medicine* 179, no. 3 (2019): 363–72.

95   **authors reported one year later:** D. M. Levine, J. A. Linder, and B. E. Landon, "Characteristics of Americans with Primary Care and Changes over Time, 2002–2015," *JAMA Internal Medicine* 180, no. 3 (2020): 463–66.

Chapter 5: Twenty-Eight Hours in Hell

102   **Being awake more than twenty-four hours:** D. Dawson and K. Reid, "Fatigue, Alcohol and Performance Impairment," *Nature* 388, no. 6639 (1997): 235; and N. Lamond and D. Dawson, "Quantifying the Performance Impairment Associated with Fatigue," *Journal of Sleep Research* 8, no. 4 (1999): 255–62.

113   **The alarm bells first rang:** R. C. Friedman, J. T. Bigger, and D. S. Kornfeld, "The Intern and Sleep Loss," *New England Journal of Medicine* 285, no. 4 (1971): 201–3.

113   **Libby Zion was just eighteen:** Barron H. Lerner. "A Life-Changing Case for Doctors in Training," *New York Times*, March 3, 2009.

114   **Her father wrote an op-ed:** Sidney Zion, "Doctors Know Best?" *New York Times*, May 13, 1989.

115   **to scour millions of hospitalizations:** A. K Rosen et al., "Effects of Resident Duty Hour Reform on Surgical and Procedural Patient Safety Indicators among Hospitalized VA and Medicare Patients," *Medical Care* 47, no. 7 (2009): 723–31.

115   **less direct patient contact:** L. Block et al., "In the Wake of the 2003 and 2011 Duty Hours Regulations, How Do Internal Medicine Interns Spend Their Time?" *Journal of General Internal Medicine* 28, no. 8 (2013): 1042–47.

115   **decreased educational opportunities:** S. V. Desai et al., "Effect of the 2011 vs 2003 Duty Hour Regulation-Compliant Models on Sleep Duration, Trainee Education, and Continuity of Patient Care among Internal Medicine House Staff: A Randomized Trial," *JAMA Internal Medicine* 173, no. 8 (2013): 649–55.

115   **only minimally increased sleep:** S. Sen et al., "Effects of the 2011 Duty Hour Reforms on Interns and Their Patients: A Prospec-

tive Longitudinal Cohort Study," *JAMA Internal Medicine* 173, no. 8 (2013): 657–62.

116 **When the results were tallied:** K. Y. Bilimoria et al., "National Cluster-Randomized Trial of Duty-Hour Flexibility in Surgical Training," *New England Journal of Medicine* 374 (2016): 713–27.

116 **a parody published:** G. C. Smith and J. P. Pell, "Parachute Use to Prevent Death and Major Trauma Related to Gravitational Challenge: Systematic Review of Randomised Controlled Trials," *British Medical Journal* 327, no. 7429 (2003): 1459–61.

118 **asked for an investigation:** Public Citizen, "iCOMPARE and FIRST Trials Comparing Standard and Long Work Schedules for Medical Residents," n.d., https://www.citizen.org/article/icompare -and-first-trials-comparing-standard-and-long-work-schedules-for -medical-residents/.

118 **"no more than minimal risk":** Protocol for S. V. Desai, D. A. Asch, L. M. Bellini, et al., "Education Outcomes in a Duty-Hour Flexibility Trial in Internal Medicine," *New England Journal of Medicine* 328 (2018): 1494–508 (supplementary appendix), available at https://www.nejm.org/doi/suppl/10.1056/NEJMoa1800965/suppl_ file/nejmoa1800965_protocol.pdf.

118 **the residency programs themselves:** L. Shepherd and R. Macklin, "Erosion of Informed Consent in U.S. Research," *Bioethics* 33, no. 1 (2019): 4–12.

119 **iCOMPARE showed:** J. H. Silber et al., "Patient Safety Outcomes under Flexible and Standard Resident Duty-Hour Rules," *New England Journal of Medicine* 380, no. 10 (2019): 905–14.

119 **doctors' well-being suffered:** S. V. Desai et al., "Education Outcomes in a Duty-Hour Flexibility Trial in Internal Medicine," *New England Journal of Medicine* 378 (2018): 1494–508.

120 **They cited an editorial:** L. Rosenbaum and D. Lamas, "Eyes Wide Open—Examining the Data on Duty-Hour Reform," *New England Journal of Medicine* 380 (2019): 969–70.

122 **In the *New York Times*:** Gina Kolata and Jan Hoffman, "New Guideline Will Allow First-Year Doctors to Work 24-Hour Shifts," *New York Times*, March 10, 2017.

Chapter 6: Reinventing Primary Care

128 **As of 2019:** K. D. Miller et al., "Cancer Treatment and Survivorship Statistics, 2019," *CA: A Cancer Journal for Clinicians* 69, no. 5 (2019): 363–85.

128 **projected to reach:** S. M. Bluethmann, A. B. Mariotto, and J. H. Rowland, "Anticipating the 'Silver Tsunami': Prevalence Trajectories and Comorbidity Burden among Older Cancer Survivors in the United States," *Cancer Epidemiology, Biomarkers & Prevention* 25, no. 7 (2016): 1029–36.

128 **one quote stopped me:** E. Grunfeld and C. C. Earle, "The Interface between Primary and Oncology Specialty Care: Treatment through Survivorship," *Journal of the National Cancer Institute: Monographs* 2010, no. 40 (2010): 25–30.

130 **predict a shortage:** IHS Markit Ltd., *The Complexities of Physician Supply and Demand: Projections from 2019 to 2034* (Washington, DC: Association of American Medical Colleges, June 2021).

131 **"The administrative burden":** Monique Tello, interview by Ilana Yurkiewicz, October 1, 2021.

132 **"You're a factory worker":** Dana Corriel, interview by Ilana Yurkiewicz, September 30, 2021.

135 **88 percent of medical care:** Apoorva Rama, "Payment and Delivery in 2020: Fee-for-Service Revenue Remains Stable While Participation Shifts in Accountable Care Organizations during the Pandemic," Policy Research Perspectives, American Medical Association, Chicago, 2021.

135 **One way it did this was:** Atul Gawande, "Overkill," *The New Yorker*, May 11, 2015.

136 **than any other outpatient specialty:** L. S. Rotenstein et al., "Differences in Total and After-Hours Electronic Health Record Time across Ambulatory Specialties," *JAMA Internal Medicine* 181, no. 6 (2021): 863–65.

137 **"Our task was to disrupt things":** Alan Glaseroff, interview by Ilana Yurkiewicz, October 8, 2021.

139 **they cost the insurance plan $43,000:** Heather Boerner, "Stanford's Big Health Care Idea," *Washington Monthly,* March 19, 2017.

142 **"It was my dream":** Nancy Cuan, interview by Ilana Yurkiewicz, October 1, 2021.

142 **"I had this Oliver Twist feeling":** Kathan Vollrath, interview by Ilana Yurkiewicz, April 26, 2022.

146 **described the concept to me:** Kate Lorig, interview by Ilana Yurkiewicz, April 20, 2022.

148 **was the dominant payment model:** S. H. Zuvekas and J. W. Cohen, "Fee-for-Service, While Much Maligned, Remains the Dominant Payment Method for Physician Visits," *Health Affairs (Millwood)* 35, no. 3 (2016): 411–14.

Chapter 7: These Things Happen

175 **his hospital had dramatically reduced:** M. L. Zeidel, "Systematic Quality Improvement in Medicine: Everyone Can Do It," *Rambam Maimonides Medical Journal* 2, no. 3 (2011): e0055.

Chapter 8: The Likeliest Unlikely

188 **over one-third of the U.S. population:** K. N. Yadav et al., "Approximately One in Three US Adults Completes Any Type of Advance Directive for End-of-Life Care," *Health Affairs (Millwood)* 36, no. 7 (2017): 1244–51.

191 **New Yorker cartoon:** Teresa Burns Parkhurst, "The Knee and Upper Shin Guy," *The New Yorker*, October 14, 2019.

196 **coauthored a book:** Daniel Kahneman, Olivier Sibony, and Cass R. Sunstein, *Noise: A Flaw in Human Judgment* (New York: Little, Brown Spark, 2021).

197 **a best-selling book:** Kerry Patterson et al., *Crucial Conversations: Tools for Talking When Stakes Are High* (New York: McGraw-Hill, 2002).

Chapter 9: Fixing Fragmentation Together

205 **published a book:** James Reason, *Human Error* (New York: Cambridge University Press, 1990).

205 **The model has been criticized:** J. Larouzee and J-C. Le Coze, "Good and Bad Reasons: The Swiss Cheese Model and Its Critics," *Safety Science* 126 (2020): 104660.

206 **Others have pointed out:** Y. Li and H. Thimbleby, "Hot Cheese: A Processed Swiss Cheese Model," *Journal of the Royal College of Physicians of Edinburgh* 44, no. 2 (2014): 116–21.

206 **Reason himself has acknowledged:** James Reason, "Überlingen: Is Swiss Cheese Past Its Sell-By Date?" Eurocontrol Experimental Centre Workshop, September 7–8, 2004, Brétigny, France.

212 **One often-cited study:** N. A. Christakis and E. B. Lamont, "Extent and Determinants of Error in Doctors' Prognoses in Terminally Ill Patients: Prospective Cohort Study," *British Medical Journal* 320, no. 7233 (2000): 469–72.

212 **56 percent of the time:** B. Gwilliam et al., "Prognosticating in Patients with Advanced Cancer: Observational Study Comparing

the Accuracy of Clinicians' and Patients' Estimates of Survival," *Annals of Oncology* 24, no. 2 (2013): 482–88.

214 **"Now, instead of wondering why":** Paul Kalanithi, *When Breath Becomes Air* (New York: Random House, 2016).

220 **wrote a powerful account:** A. E. Caruso Brown, "Porous Boundaries," *Journal of the American Medical Association* 317, no. 24 (2017): 2487–88.

221 **"necessary collusion":** P. R. Helft, "Necessary Collusion: Prognostic Communication with Advanced Cancer Patients," *Journal of Clinical Oncology* 23, no. 13 (2005): 3146–50.

225 **debunked the waste theory:** L. Einav et al., "Predictive Modeling of U.S. Health Care Spending in Late Life," *Science* 360, no. 6396 (2018): 1462–65.

Index